A Commonwealth Response to a Global Health Challenge

COMMONWEALTH SECRETARIAT

Commonwealth Secretariat
Marlborough House
Pall Mall, London SW1Y 5HX
United Kingdom

Published by the Commonwealth Secretariat
Printed in the United Kingdom by Formara Ltd

Wherever possible, the Commonwealth Secretariat uses paper sourced
from sustainable forests or from sources that minimise a destructive impact
on the environment.

Price: £8.99

ISBN: 0-85092-651-3

Web site:
http://www.thecommonwealth.org

Contents

Preface

Ministers of Health at their thirty-fourth annual meeting prior to the World Health Assembly in Geneva on 13 May 2001 welcomed the increasing attention being given to HIV/AIDS at high-level international fora. They noted with satisfaction the efforts being made in the Commonwealth to ensure that the strength, impact and visibility of the Commonwealth's collective response to the pandemic is maximised. They were also very pleased with the intensive regional efforts that have been taking place across the Commonwealth, including the development of regional strategies in Africa, Asia and the Caribbean.

The Commonwealth Secretariat is also engaged in activities relating to many of the areas identified in the UN Declaration of Commitment on HIV/AIDS adopted on 27 June 2001. The Secretariat is reviewing the Declaration to identify areas for continued expanded action and possible new niche areas. In particular, it will intensify its partnerships with Commonwealth non-governmental organisations, development agencies and other partners to assist member states to tackle the increasing burden of the HIV/AIDS pandemic.

Over the past year, the Secretariat has been involved in a number of initiatives. These include the setting up of an Inter-Divisional Task Force on HIV/AIDS that meets regularly to review the work of the Secretariat on AIDS; the preparation of expert papers for ministerial meetings on finance, health, women and youth to create awareness of HIV/AIDS among ministers; promotion of a Youth as Ambassadors for Positive Living Programme; development of AIDS fact sheets for Secretariat staff and consultants; and production of a pamphlet on HIV/AIDS as a gender issue.

This publication, *A Commonwealth Response to a Global Health Challenge*, incorporates many strategies for HIV/AIDS prevention and treatment, and is a means of sharing experiences and lessons from around the Commonwealth. The articles it contains provide information on the prevention and treatment of HIV/AIDS, and also encourage a positive outlook and give hope for the future.

HIV/AIDS:
Prevention and Care

Care for People Living with HIV/AIDS*

Elly Katabira, Francis Mubiru and Eric van Praag

John found out he was HIV-positive in 1989 when he was offered a university place in the USA. Before he took up his place he was required to undergo a medical examination which included an HIV test. He was devastated when the positive result came back. Not only had he lost the opportunity of studying abroad but he also had to face the knowledge that he had a terminal illness which he could not talk about and for which there was very little hope of treatment.

Eventually he went to the city's hospital where a small HIV clinic was run by a non-governmental organisation (NGO), and he took up a counselling course as a volunteer. After some months he felt able to use his skills to help others learn about HIV. Over the following years he visited numerous schools, workplaces and clinics to talk about HIV and use his personal experience to educate others and destigmatise this condition. He remained well until 1994, when he developed tuberculosis. This was successfully treated and he was able to return to work. His health deteriorated again in late 1995, and he had a bout of pneumonia and recurrent abscesses. He continued to be active in the People Living with HIV/AIDS (PLHA) network and was always very well informed about the latest developments in HIV treatments, particularly the new antiretroviral treatments (ARV). When he arranged a PLHA meeting to discuss ARVs, not a single person at the meeting was using ARVs or had any likelihood of ever doing so.

John's health then deteriorated and he had to stop work. Despite having given more than seven years of his life to educating people about HIV, he died in poverty – unable during the last few months to buy all the food he needed, let alone any medication.

Support Urgently Needed

John's case illustrates the prolonged and devastating effects that HIV infection and AIDS have at a personal level. It also highlights some of the new approaches that health services and communities have developed to meet the various needs of people living with HIV/AIDS, such as counselling and support groups. It also shows that some of the successful drug interventions in parts of the industrialised world are just a dream in many other settings.

People living with HIV/AIDS have a variety of needs and problems related to their condition. It is essential to appreciate and understand these needs in order to develop practical, realistic and achievable care. In most countries, HIV infection

*This material was first published in *World Health*, November–December 1998.

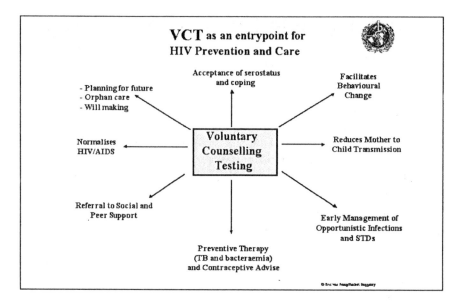

predominantly affects young people in their most productive period of life. Ultimately fatal, it may last for many years with episodes of illnesses that alternate with disease-free periods. The infection further provokes strong emotional reactions which lead to stigmatisation and rejection not only by communities but even by health staff, even though the disease has been around for almost 20 years. Care responses have to be very wide in order to cover such needs as clinical, nursing, psychological and social support. These responses have developed in many countries, particularly in Africa, faced with an escalating HIV epidemic. Initiatives have come from a variety of sources, including PLHA themselves and their affected relatives and friends, from NGOs and from various support groups organised at community, hospital or national level. Comprehensive care responds to medical, emotional and social needs.

A Care Continuum

A synthesis of these approaches, based on lessons learned so far, resulted in the concept of comprehensive care across a continuum. This recognises the need for care through all stages of HIV infection, which should be accessible at several points along a continuum from voluntary testing, counselling sites and hospital and social services, to community-based support groups and home-based care.

A good example of such an approach is The AIDS Support Organisation (TASO) in Uganda. Several government health workers and affected relatives of HIV-infected patients established an NGO and ran weekly clinics in some national hospitals, where comprehensive care was provided. TASO provides medical services, counselling and social support for clients and their families as well as establishing linkages

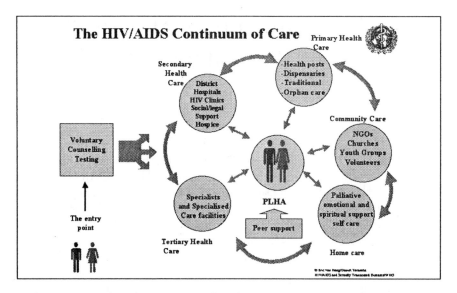

with community-based initiatives such as home care. Community workers in turn refer the client back to the TASO clinic, when necessary, for more specialised support to ensure comprehensive care across the continuum from home to hospital.

As the HIV epidemic enters a third decade, the challenge is how to expand care to ensure that PLHA have access to voluntary testing and counselling, and to the newer or improved clinical interventions, such as providing isoniazid, a cheap and widely available drug which prevents tuberculosis.

The latest addition to any continuum of care project is the introduction of antiretroviral drugs if they can be afforded. At present, ARV drugs are too expensive for the majority of HIV-infected people and, even if available, are effective only for about 50 per cent of patients. In countries with limited resources, access is further constrained by the limited number of clinicians and nurses who know how to use these drugs effectively and safely, as they very often interact with other medications. Yet if taken with appropriate monitoring and supervision, ARV therapies will prevent opportunistic infections occurring for months, or even years, and thus improve the quality of life of many patients.

For any expanded care programme to be successful, there must be voluntary counselling and testing to help people infected with HIV to know and accept their seropositive status. In this way they are able to participate fully in medical, social and psychological interventions, even in an environment which is often not conducive to compliance. Joint efforts are being made, involving the people affected, clinical and research institutions, the donor community, and agencies such as UNAIDS, UNICEF and the World Health Organisation (WHO). They are seeking to respond to the challenges in the most severely affected countries, and are widely promoting initiatives such as TASO.

5

Lessons Learned from AIDS Health Promotion

John Hubley

With formidable obstacles to be overcome before treatment becomes effective, affordable and universally available, prevention through the adoption of safer sexual behaviours remains the most important strategy for tackling the AIDS epidemic. At the Leeds Health Education Database Project, we have been developing a database of evaluated health promotion interventions from the developing world. Of the 342 published programmes in this database, 52 are for health promotion interventions for AIDS and STDs in the Commonwealth. This is the largest single group of interventions represented – a tribute to the global effort directed at tackling the AIDS epidemic. A selection are reviewed below. I have given priority to recent interventions that provide statistically significant evidence of impact, and a spread of target group, methodology and country.

Clinic-based health promotion, including counselling, is a common approach for ensuring compliance with STD medication, reduction in demand for injections, ensuring return for follow-up treatment and adoption of risk-reduction behaviour including the use of condoms. People with STDs are a section of the community who are at potential risk of HIV both through their lifestyle and through the STD itself. One of the most important findings of the last decade was the demonstration in the Mwanza study in Tanzania that treatment and counselling STD patients could reduce transmission of HIV. Some of the early evaluations had demonstrated the limitations of advice given during a single encounter with the patient. More success has been found with advice that is reinforced with follow-up visits and supported with well-designed and pre-tested educational materials and that involves participatory methods. A challenge is to break down barriers between family planning and STD programmes to create an integrated approach to reproductive and sexual health.

However, effective AIDS health promotion must go out of the health facility into the community. Examples from Uganda show the power of community-based approaches to influence practices. Religion is often mistakenly perceived as a barrier to health promotion activities. The benefits of working through religious leaders was shown by an evaluation of a programme working with Imams in Uganda.

Folk media based on oral traditions, including drama, music and puppetry, have an important potential through their emotional impact and entertainment value. Evaluations demonstrate their power to attract large audiences, provide knowledge and encourage community participation. Drama is a particularly useful tool to use in working with local communities or schools and there are good examples of its use from South Africa, India and Sri Lanka. While effective in reaching communities, there are costs and logistical problems involved in sustaining a full-time theatre group for AIDS education. Larger numbers of people can be reached by broadcasting drama on mass media.

Mass media, especially radio, have been effectively used to reach large numbers of people. They can be used on their own or as part of a condom social marketing programme. Published evaluations from Tanzania, Zambia, St Vincent and the Grenadines, and St Lucia demonstrate that mass media can be effective in conveying information, influencing attitudes and possibly behaviour change if care is taken in choosing the content so that it is relevant, interesting and understandable to the intended audience and if the material is pre-tested before it is broadcast. A good approach is to plan the content and timing of mass media to support and reinforce face-to-face work by field staff.

These programmes need to be complemented by health promotion targeted at specific groups who are themselves at risk or who may be a risk to others. Prostitutes, also called sex workers, may work full time or on an occasional basis from bars, brothels or on the street in towns, cities and along road transport routes. One of the first success stories in AIDS programmes was the demonstration that educational activities carried out with prostitutes in Nairobi could reduce their rate of HIV infection. This early programme has been followed up by reports of successful programmes with female prostitutes and male transsexuals in Nigeria, Malawi, India and Singapore. The impact demonstrated includes improved ability to negotiate safe sex with clients, increased condom use and reduced incidence of STDs. These evaluations have raised some important issues. Sex workers are a marginalised section of the community and educational methods need to go beyond just providing information, to empower them with the skills and confidence to negotiate safer sex with clients. The more successful programmes have used participatory approaches including the selection and training of sex workers as peer educators, and combined this with providing condoms, treating STDs and supportive counselling. It is also important that the sex worker is not blamed for the problem. Educational programmes also have to be directed to the clients of sex workers. Programmes targeting sex workers should address the economic reasons why women take up sex work and also provide support in finding alternative ways of generating income. It is often necessary to introduce legal measures to reduce victimisation, police harassment and discrimination.

Other targeted programmes are also necessary. Intensive programmes are now underway to reach men who travel away from home, especially truck drivers. In Kenya, a creative mix of educational activities at transport companies and roadside halts, and specialist clinics resulted in a decrease of STDs and a reduction in sexual risk behaviours. Peer group education methods were effective in increasing knowledge about AIDS and condom use among truck drivers in Tanzania. In India, evaluations have been able to demonstrate impacts on a section of the community

7

that has been difficult to reach – injecting drug users. In Mozambique, evaluations have demonstrated an impact on prisoners, another section of the community who are especially at risk.

Schools are one of the most important ways of reaching young persons before they begin sexual activity. Evaluated interventions have demonstrated that it is not difficult to improve the knowledge of pupils about AIDS, but that it is more difficult to influence practice. One-off sessions by external speakers do not have a lasting impact on attitudes and behaviour change. However, good examples exist from Uganda, Malawi and South Africa of programmes which have used participatory methods and a life-skills decision-making approach, provided training for teachers, involved parents and carried out longer-term interventions integrated within the broader school curriculum. These have demonstrated that it is possible to influence pupils' stated intentions towards sex in some cases. Unfortunately, these evaluations also show the formidable obstacles ahead. Lack of training and support for teachers, large classes and poorly equipped schools make it difficult for many schools to implement the kind of AIDS education that is needed to have an impact on the problem.

Approaches in school need to be complemented by out-of-school approaches which can reach non-attenders including early drop-outs and street children. An approach that has been widely adopted is selecting and training young people to provide education among their peers – an example of this approach is cited below from Sri Lanka.

As we enter the new century we can point with confidence at evidence from evaluated studies that well-planned health promotion can bring about increases in knowledge, skills, attitudes, change in behaviour and, in some cases, health status. Successful health promotion comes from the systematic and planned application of a combination of measures including basing the programme on an understanding of the community, for example through baseline research, defining the intended targets, using participatory approaches, and providing training and support for field staff and health care providers. These need to be carried out alongside the development of supportive environments including health and other services adequately staffed with trained and supportive staff; a multisectoral approach involving governmental and non-governmental bodies in health, education, economic, employment and legal affairs; a gender-sensitive approach which addresses the distinct needs of both women and men; and fostering a legal environment which protects against discrimination. We now know how to prevent AIDS. The challenge is to put this knowledge into practice.

Bibliography

Some evaluated interventions from the Leeds Health Education Database

Clinic-based education and counselling for AIDS/STD control

Grosskurth, H, Mosha, F, Todd, J, Mwijarubi, E, Klokke, A, Senkoro, K, Mayaud, P, Changalucha, J, Nicoll, A and ka-Gina, G (1995). 'Impact of improved treatment of sexually transmitted diseases on HIV infection in rural Tanzania: randomised controlled trial' (Mwanza study).

Pickering, H, Quigley, M, Pepin, J, Todd, J and Wilkins, A (1993). 'The effects of post-test counselling on condom use among prostitutes in The Gambia', *AIDS* 7, 271–3.

Wilkins, HA, Alonso, P, Baldeh, S, Cham, MK, Corrah, T, Hughes, A, Jaiteh, KO, Oelman, B and Pickering, H (1989). 'Knowledge of AIDS, use of condoms and results of counselling subjects with asymptomatic HIV2 infection in The Gambia', *AIDS Care* 1, 247–56.

General community programmes

Kagimu, M, Marum, E, Nakyanjo, N, Walakir, Y and Hogle, J (1998). 'Evaluation of the effectiveness of AIDS health education interventions in the Muslim community in Uganda', *AIDS Education and Prevention* 10(3): 215–28.

Schopper, D, Doussantousse, S, Ayiga, N, Ezatirale, G, Idro, WJ and Homsy, J (1995). 'Village-Based AIDS Prevention in a Rural District in Uganda', *Health Policy and Planning* (2): 171–80.

Popular media including drama and music

McGill, D and Joseph, WD (1997). 'An HIV/AIDS awareness prevention project in Sri Lanka: evaluation of drama and flyer distribution interventions', *International Quarterly of Community Health Education* 16, 237–55.

Skinner, D, Metcalf, CA, Seager, JR, de-Swardt, JS et al (1991). 'An evaluation of an education programme on HIV infection using puppetry and street theatre. Special Section: AIDS – the first ten years', *AIDS Care* 3(3): 317–29.

Valente, TW and Bharath, U (1999). 'An evaluation of the use of drama to communicated HIV/AIDS information', *AIDS Education and Prevention* 11, 203–11.

Mass media

Middlestadt, S, Fishbein, M, Albarracin, D, Francis, C, Eustace, MA, Helquist, M and Schneider, A (1995). 'Evaluating the impact of a national AIDS prevention radio campaign in St Vincent and the Grenadines', *Journal of Applied Social Psychology* 25, 21–34. Ref ID: 8477.

Vaughan, PW, Regis, A and St Catherine, E (2000). 'Effects of an entertainment-education radio soap opera on family planning and HIV prevention in St Lucia', *International Family Planning Perspectives* 26, 148–57.

Yoder, PS, Hornik, R and Chirwa, BC (1996). 'Evaluating the program effects of a radio drama about AIDS in Zambia', *Studies in Family Planning* 27(4): 188–203.

Targeted interpersonal interventions directed at sex workers

Asamoah-Adu, A, Weir, S, Pappoe, M, Kanlisi, N, Neequaye, A and Lamptey, P (1994). 'Evaluation of a targeted AIDS prevention intervention to increase condom use among prostitutes in Ghana', AIDS 8(2): 239–46.

Asthana, S and Oostvogels, R (1996). 'Community Participation in HIV Prevention: Problems and Prospects for Community-Based Strategies among Female Sex Workers in Madras, India', Social Science and Medicine 43, 133–48.

Bhave, G, Lindan, C P, Hudes, E S, Desai, S, Wagle, U, Tripathi, S P and Mandel, J S (1995). 'Impact of an intervention on HIV, sexually transmitted diseases, and condom use among sex workers in Bombay, India', AIDS 9 Suppl 1, S21–30.

Esu-Williams, E (1998). 'Sexually transmitted diseases and condom interventions among prostitutes and their clients in Cross River State Nigeria', Health Transition Review 5, 223–8.

Moses, S, Plummer, F A, Ngugi, E N, Nagelkerke, N J, Anzala, A O and Ndinya-Achola, J (1991). 'Controlling HIV in Africa: Effectiveness and cost of an intervention in a high-frequency STD transmitter core group (Kenya)', AIDS 5, 407–11.

Walden, V M, Mwangulube, K and Makhumula-Nkhoma, P (1999). 'Measuring the impact of a behaviour change intervention for commercial sex workers and their potential clients in Malawi', Health Education Research: Theory and Practice 14, 545–54.

Wong, M L, Chan, K W and Koh, D (1998). 'A sustainable behavioural intervention to increase condom use and reduce gonorrhea among sex workers in Singapore: 2-year follow-up', Preventive Medicine 27, 891–900. Ref ID: 8398.

Other targeted programmes

Vaz, R G, Gloyd, S and Trinidade, R (1996). 'The effects of peer education on STD and AIDS knowledge among prisoners in Mozambique', International Journal of STD and AIDS 7, 51–4.

Hangzo, C, Chatterjee, A, Sarkar, S, Zomi, G T, Deb, B C and Abdul-Quader, A S (1997). 'Reaching out beyond the hills: HIV prevention among injecting drug users in Manipur, India', Addiction 92(7): 813–20.

Jackson, D J, Rakwar, J P, Richardson, B A, Mandliya, K, Chohan, B H, Bwayo, J J, Ndinya-Achola, J O, Martin, H L, Moses, S and Kreiss, J K (1997). 'Decreased incidence of sexually transmitted diseases among trucking company workers in Kenya: results of a behavioural risk-reduction programme', AIDS 11, 903–9.

Laukamm-Josten, U, Mwizarubi, B K, Outwater, A, Mwaijonga, C L, Valadez, J J, Nyamwaya, D, Swai, R, Saidel, T and Nyamuryekunge'e K (2000). 'Preventing HIV infection through peer education and condom promotion among truck drivers and their sexual partners in Tanzania, 1990–1993', AIDS Care 12, 27–40.

Cameron, K A, Witte, K, Lapinski, M K and Nzyuko, S (1998). 'Preventing HIV transmission along the Trans-Africa Highway in Kenya: using persuasive message theory in formative education', International Quarterly of Community Health Education 18, 331–56.

School-based and youth-targeted programmes for HIV/AIDS/reproductive health

Awasthi, S, Nichter, M and Pande, V K (2000). 'Developing an interactive STD-prevention programme for youth: lessons from a North Indian slum', *Stud. Fam. Plann.* 31, 138–50.

Dalrymple, L and du-Toit, M K (1993). 'The evaluation of a drama approach to AIDS education', *Educational Psychology* 13(2): 147–54.

Fitzgerald, A M, Stanton, B F, Terreri, N, Shipena, H, Li, X, Kahihuata, J, Ricardo, I B, Galbraith, J S and De Jaeger, A M (1999). 'Use of Western-based HIV risk-reduction interventions targeting adolescents in an African setting', *Journal of Adolescent Health* 25, 52–61.

Kinsman, J, Nakiyingi, J K A, Carpenter, L Q M P R and Whitworth, J (2001). 'Evaluation of a comprehensive school-based AIDS education programme in rural Masaka, Uganda', *Health Education Research: Theory and Practice* 16, 85–100.

Klepp, K I, Ndeki, S S, Seha, A M, Hannan, P, Lyimo B A, Msuya, M H, Irema, M N and Schreiner, A (1994). 'AIDS education for primary school children in Tanzania: an evaluation study', *AIDS* 1157–62.

Kuhn, L, Steinberg, M and Mathews, C (1994). 'Participation of the school community in AIDS education: an evaluation of a high school programme in South Africa', *AIDS Care* 6(2): 161–71, .

MacLachlan, M, Chimombo, M and Mpemba, N (1997). 'AIDS education for youth through active learning: a school-based approach from Malawi', *International Journal of Educational Development* 17, 41–50.

Nastasi, B, Schensul, J J, Amarasiri de Silfa, M W, Varjas, K, Silva, K T, Ratnayake, P and Schensul, S (1998). 'Community-based sexual risk prevention programme for Sri Lankan youth: influencing sexual-risk decision making', *International Quarterly of Community Health Education* 18, 139–55.

Shuey, D A, Babishangire, B B, Omiat, S and Bagarukayo, H. (1999). 'Increased sexual abstinence among school adolescents as a result of school health education in Soroti district, Uganda', *Health Education Research: Theory and Practice* 14, 411–19.

A full listing is available on request of all the interventions on AIDS in the Leeds Health Education Database.

Health Promotion and Health Education and HIV/AIDS

Margaret Sills

Summary

An outline of the principles of health promotion based on the Ottawa Charter (1986) and the Jakarta Declaration (1997) is offered as a reminder of the nature of an approach that can span sectors in a multi-disciplinary way. This is essential in the efforts to control HIV transmission and AIDS-related illnesses.

The school setting is then taken as an example, and a range of effective methods and approaches focusing on young people is identified. Finally, a brief consideration of monitoring health status is offered.

Introduction

It is clear that the prevention and treatment of HIV/AIDS is not exclusively a health or medical problem. HIV and AIDS-related illnesses are having a considerable impact on the social and economic structures of many societies. This points to the need for policies and action across all sectors and at all levels of government if the epidemic is to be reversed; the mainstreaming of health has never been more urgent.

This article will focus on the role that health promotion can play in preventing the transmission of HIV (the nature, incidence and prevalence of HIV and AIDS-related illnesses are comprehensively dealt with elsewhere). An outline of the nature of health promotion will be followed by consideration of school-based efforts, which aim to protect the future generation, and a summary of some of the strategies that have been effective in this setting. Finally, issues related to health and monitoring health status are then very briefly addressed.

Principles of Health Promotion in Relation to HIV/AIDS

The determinants of health are wide ranging and are increasingly identified with structural/societal factors as well as with personal lifestyle. Approaches to health sytems and health care systems across the Commonwealth are being reformed and reoriented from a curative and disease treatment approach to an approach which embraces prevention and health promotion to a greater degree than in the recent past. The major determinants of health, and more specifically of HIV and AIDS, are social and economic; this reinforces the need to look further than the health sector in order to make improvements effectively.

Health promotion is a process of enabling individuals and communities to live their lives to the full, as well as avoiding illness and preventable disability, through strengthening their capacity to control, improve and maintain their health as a resource for everyday life. Health promotion specialists are in a position to create bridges and support a multisectoral approach. However, everyone has a responsibility to ensure that their actions promote rather than demote health.

There is clear evidence (WHO, 1998) that comprehensive approaches which use combinations of the following five strategies (Ottawa Charter, 1986) are the most effective:

- building healthy public policy;[1]
- creating supportive environments;
- strengthening community action;
- developing personal skills;
- reorienting health services towards promotion and prevention.

There is also evidence (WHO, 1998) that:

- certain settings offer practical opportunities for the implementation of comprehensive strategies, such as cities, islands, local communities, markets, schools, workplaces and health services;
- people have to be put at the centre of health promotion action and decision-making processes if these are to be effective;
- access to education and information is vital in achieving effective participation and the empowerment of people and communities;
- health promotion is a 'key investment' and an essential element of health development.

In 1997 the Jakarta Declaration (WHO) identified five global priorities for health promotion in the twenty-first century, all of which are pertinent to the HIV/AIDS predicament that the Commonwealth now faces:

- *Promote social responsibility for health:* public and private sector decision-makers should pursue policies and practices that are committed to social responsibility and include equity-focused health impact assessments as an integral part of policy development. Assessment data should be disaggregated for essential indicators including gender and age.

- *Increase investments for health development:* this requires a truly multisectoral approach, including, for example, increasing or reorientating existing resources in education and housing as well as for the health sector. The needs of poor and marginalised populations must be reflected; this is where the highest prevalence of HIV is located.

- *Consolidate and expand partnerships for health:* sharing expertise, skills and resources is mutually beneficial. Partnerships must be transparent, accountable and based on agreed ethical principles, mutual understanding and respect.

- *Increase community capacity and empower the individual:* health promotion is carried out by and with people, not on, for, or to people. It improves both the ability of individuals to take action and the capacity of groups, organisations or communities to influence their health determinants.

- *Secure an infrastructure for health promotion:* new mechanisms of funding must be found to support the basic infrastructure built on the foundations of a 'settings for health' approach.

The World Health Assembly resolution (May 1998) confirmed the priorities set out in the Jakarta declaration and urged all member states to:

- Promote social responsibility for health;

- Increase investments for health development;

- Consolidate and expand partnerships for health;

- Increase community capacity and empower the individual in matters of health;

- Strengthen consideration of health requirements and promotion in all policies;

- Adopt an evidence-based approach to health promotion policy and practice, using the full range of quantitative and qualitative methodologies.

These principles underpin the health promotion approach to combating HIV and AIDS-related illnesses.

The process of health promotion is generally thought to be most effective if it starts at the community level; indeed, there is some convincing evidence, for example from the work of Paulo Friere (1972) who encourages the consideration of the advantages of a problem-posing education in which learners become co-investigators with the facilitator. Friere saw people as subjects of transforming actions, not simply objects of action which is oppressive. An appropriate, non-oppressive form of education would be empowerment education which encourages people to be active rather than passive in person-centred learning and planning. As Wallerstein et al (1998) describe:

[I]t involves people in group efforts to identify their problems, to critically assess social and historical roots of problems, to envision a healthier society, and to develop strategies to overcome obstacles in achieving their goals.

Behavioural intervention programmes can be effective. In Mombasa, Kenya, for example, 556 male HIV seronegative employees of a trucking company were offered a behavioural intervention programme and free condoms aiming to reduce the incidence of high-risk sexual behaviour and the incidence of STDs declined

(Jackson et al, 1997). Zambia and Kenya (Yoder, 1996) have used radio soap operas with some success in meeting the challenges of AIDS education. However, while marketing and the power of radio and television may be useful in disseminating information and playing a supportive role, health information must not be confused with health education (McDonald, 1993).

The next section looks at health promotion, health education and HIV/AIDS related issues arising in the school setting where efforts to protect the future generations are concentrated.

Health Promotion and Health Education in Schools

As Ellis and Figuera (1998) remind us, practitioners in school systems are not only relating to students with HIV/AIDS and the associated physiological ramifications but also dealing with:

• prevention

• education

• dissemination of information

• skill development

• elimination of risk in a case of emergency

• assuaging fears and anxieties of parents, teachers, students and the community

• provision of social support

• referrals to appropriate practitioners

• advocating appropriate policy development.

Appropriate training and capacity building in health promotion and health education are required in general, but more specifically the attitudes, skills and knowledge required to address HIV/AIDS related issues are crucial. Resources such as those produced by WHO/UNESCO (Robertson, 1994) and UTA (Bhagbanprakash, 1993) may be useful.

As is well documented elsewhere, the main risk behaviours leading to the transmission of HIV are sexual intercourse (anal, vaginal and oral), sharing needles whilst injecting drugs, and exposure to blood and blood products, as well as tattooing, body piercing with unsterilised needles and shaving with unsterilised razors. Many factors contribute to increasing the incidence of these risk behaviours, particularly in young people, such as:

• low educational attainment

• use of alcohol

- use of non-injecting drugs

- homelessness

- mental health difficulties

- low self-esteem

- poverty

- sexual molestation and rape

- anything that contributes to the disenfranchisement of youth.

These can be considered as indirect factors but are nevertheless very useful indicators for health promotion interventions. Risk reduction techniques are an important corollary to reducing HIV transmission.

Labonté (1998) reminds us that most risk conditions are unequally distributed by virtue of being conditions of comparative inequality. It is not possible to have low status without high status or poverty without wealth. People who experience low status and poverty have more disease and less well-being. Health status rises with social status and the concomitant power and wealth. The greater the relative distribution of power and wealth, the greater the difference in health status between top and bottom. HIV/AIDS is no exception to this.

Ameliorating the Severity and Spread of HIV/AIDS through Health Promotion

What Works with Young People?

Life Skills programmes are important and are successful when they use participatory methods and experiential learning techniques, and when they are addressed in specific lessons rather than being spread throughout the curriculum (Gachuhi, 1999).

It is impossible to say that a particular strategy will work in all cultures and situations. However, Ellis and Figuera (1998) summarise a review of the literature which suggests that the following health promotion and health education programme approaches can be effective in HIV prevention with young people. Some of the main points are:

- Education and interventions that are culturally and linguistically appropriate and specifically tailored to the appropriate literacy level;

- Frank and open discussion regarding the risks of unprotected sexual activity (in a safe environment);

- Sexual negotiation and role playing strategies that actively engage the participants in discussion, free thinking and problem solving;

- Accurate and careful instruction regarding the use of condoms and needle cleansing;
- Frank and open discussion regarding the benefits of both sexual and chemical abstinence;
- Chemical dependency and treatment programmes designed specifically for target populations, for example adolescents;
- Needle exchange and sterilisation programmes for young people with chemical dependency;
- Programmes that provide housing, education, and opportunities for under-privileged youth;
- Community based programmes that link schools with community-based prevention activities;
- Use of HIV seropositive and seronegative peer educators in the classroom setting;
- Street outreach programmes involving peer education, promotion of condom use and distribution;
- Readily available HIV testing services designed specifically for adolescent populations;
- Frank and open discussion regarding homophobia, sexual orientation and the risk of heterosexual transmission for women and children;
- Social marketing strategies that make safer sex negotiation and abstinence socially desirable;
- Programmes that include extensive discussion regarding the difference between contraceptive methods and their ability to prevent pregnancy versus HIV and STDs;
- Programme development that focuses on adolescent decision-making, organisation and empowerment;
- Programmes that emphasise changing group and social norms;
- Programmes that increase self efficacy and sexual efficacy among adolescents.

It is now common understanding that knowledge and information alone are unlikely to lead to changes in behaviour and must be accompanied by values clarification, attitude review and skill development. Knowledge must be taught in a practical setting that emphasises hands-on learning techniques as much as possible. Simultaneous instruction on how to use condoms with distribution of condoms and the recognition of the benefits that will come from widespread changes in condom-related behavioural norms will promote the long-term behavioural efficacy required to prevent HIV infection throughout an individual's sexually active life.

It is important to use both practical and strategic approaches. For example, a man uses condoms and therefore a practical approach is appropriate. However, a woman does not actually use condoms and a strategic approach must be employed to enable her to negotiate their use with her partner. Differences in gender are both social and biological and therefore approaches and programmes need to be tailored accordingly. It is not appropriate to assume that 'one size fits all' and that the same approach is equally appropriate to the needs of both boys and girls, men and women.

Theoretical approaches should be combined so that the multi-dimensionality of risk behaviour is retained (Ahia, 1991). Self efficacy theory (Bandura, 1992) employed in tandem with approaches from the harm reduction model will influence both an individual's behaviour and perceptions regarding their ability to change and/or carry out a particular behaviour, as well as tackling the social and environmental structures within which the behaviour occurs in order to create a climate more conducive to less risky behaviours. .

Monitoring Health Status

At the 12th Commonwealth Health Ministers' Meeting (Barbados 1998) it was agreed that Health Systems have four functions – to promote health, prevent and treat disease, and rehabilitate those with long-term chronic illnesses or disabilities. People living with HIV and AIDS-related illnesses have as much right to the best quality of life as other citizens, however they may define their health experience. The following broad categories of health experience need to be taken into account (Labonté, 1998):

• feeling vital, full of energy

• having a sense of purpose in life

• experiencing a connectedness to community

• being able to do things one enjoys

• having good social relationships

• experiencing a sense of control over one's life and living conditions.

Questions are seldom posed about people's emotional and social experiences (Bowling, 1997). Yet people's experiences of health are generally determined more by the quality of their emotional and social situations than by the absence of disease or disability (Blaxter, 1990). Monitoring of health status of those with HIV/AIDS should include subjective indicators of well-being and objective indicators of social and environmental conditions as well as the incidence and prevalence of related illnesses. It is quite possible to feel healthy whilst living with recognised disease if health or well-being and illness or disease are placed on two intersecting continua rather than at the poles of one continuum.

Conclusion

Populations, at whatever level, are diverse. Practitioners and policy-makers should diligently practice active listening, and involve the population in finding their own solutions. The choices and decisions involved are complex. There is no one right way but by working together, listening to each other and learning from other people's experiences a way forward is more likely to be found in any particular situation.

References

Ahia, R N (1991). 'Compliance with safer-sex guidelines among adolescent males: Application of the Health Belief Model and Protection Motivation Theory', *Journal of Health Education* 22(1) 49–52.

Bandura, A (1992). 'A social cognitive approach to the exercise of control over AIDS prevention'. In De Clemente, R, ed. *Adolescents and AIDS: A Generation in Jeopardy*, pp. 89–116. Newbury Park: Sage.

Bhagbanprakash, ed. (1993). *AIDS Education for student youth: A training manual*, Universities Talk AIDS (UTA), India.

Blaxter, M (1990). *Health and Lifestyles*. Routledge.

Downie, R S, Tannahill, C and Tannahill, A (1996). *Healthy Promotion: Models and Values*, 2nd edition. Oxford: Oxford University Press.

Ellis, B R and Figuera (1998). 'HIV/AIDS'. In Henderson, A C, Champlin, S and Evashwick, W, eds, *Promoting Teen Health: Linking Schools, Health Organisations and Community*, Chapter 9. Thousand Oaks: Sage Publications. ISBN: 0-76190-276-7.

Forrester, C, Thompson, P and Brandon, P (1997). 'Health Promotion'. In *Health conditions in the Caribbean*. PAHO Sci. Pub. No 561 pp.117–30.

Friere, P (1972). *Pedagogy of the Oppressed*. Penguin Books.

Gachuhi, D (1999). 'The Impact of HIV/AIDS on Education Systems in the Eastern and Southern African Region and the Response of Education Systems to HIV/AIDS: Life Skills Programmes'. UNICEF presentation at the All Sub-Saharan Africa conference on EFA 2000, 6–10 December 1999, Johannesburg, South Africa.

Jackson, D J et al (1997). 'Decrease incidence of sexually transmitted disease amongst trucking company workers in Kenya: results of a behavioural risk-reduction programme', *AIDS* 903–9.

Labonté, R (1998). 'Improving health status, quality of life and equity of access: Cultural perceptions of health and well-being, and health promotion'. Commonwealth Health Ministers Meeting, Background Paper HMM(98)(CB)2.

McDonald, J (1993). *Primary Health Care: Medicine in its Place.* Earthscan Publications Ltd, London.

Robertson, A (1994). *School Health Education to prevent AIDS and STD.* WHO/UNESCO.

Wallerstein, N and Bernstein, E (1988). 'Empowerment Education: Friere's Ideas Adapted to Health Education', *Health Education Quarterly* 15(4) pp. 379–94.

World Health Organisation (1997). *The Jakarta Declaration on Leading Health Promotion into the 21st Century.* Geneva: WHO.

World Health Organisation (1998). Health Promotion, Fifty-first World Health Assembly. (51.12) 16 May 1998.

Yoder, P S (1996). *Evaluating the programme effects of a radio drama about AIDS in Zambia.*

Note

1. Forrester et al (1997), in an article on 'Health Promotion in the Caribbean', remind us that: 'Formulating Healthy Public Policy has been variously construed. In practice, it appears to be understood mainly as constructing public health policies rather than addressing the impact of public policies on health. However, healthy public policy is not the same thing as public health policy. To say this is not to devalue the importance of public health policies but merely to recognise that all public policies have health implications.'

Issues Involved with HIV Vaccines

José Esparza and Winnie K. Mpanju-Shumbusho

Twenty years ago no-one could have suspected that a new pathogen was silently spreading in the human population. That pathogen is the human immunodeficiency virus (HIV), the etiological agent of AIDS, a disease that was first described in 1981. Over this short period of time, HIV/AIDS has become the most important infectious disease, the first cause of death in Africa and the fourth worldwide.

Early in the epidemic we learned how the virus is transmitted. With time we also defined the social context that increases risk or vulnerability to HIV infection. With that information, the international community mounted an energetic response against HIV/AIDS. There is no doubt that this rapid response was instrumental in slowing the progress of the epidemic, especially in selected populations in the industrialised world. Unfortunately, the virus continues to spread at a rate of 15,000 new infections every day, most of them occurring in developing countries.

The explanation for this situation could be twofold. Because of logistical and/or financial limitations, we are not applying, to the fullest extent possible, the health promotion interventions that we know to work (including safe blood, behavioural change, condom use, early diagnosis and treatment of STDs, etc.). On the other hand, we may still need to develop or improve additional prevention tools, including microbicides, antiretroviral drugs to prevent vertical mother-to-child transmission and vaccines.

An HIV Vaccine is Urgently Needed

As is the case with other infectious diseases, a safe, highly effective and affordable preventive vaccine may be the best long-term hope for controlling the HIV/AIDS pandemic, especially in developing countries. And we say 'long-term hope' because the development of an HIV vaccine will not be easy, nor will it be quickly found. Moreover, even when a vaccine is developed, it will not completely replace other preventive interventions, especially if the first generation of HIV vaccines only show moderate efficacy. It is more likely that an HIV vaccine will have to be delivered as part of a comprehensive prevention package, with the appropriate interventions being applied to the appropriate populations, in a 'mixture' defined through epidemiological, social/behavioural and operational research.

An HIV Vaccine is Possible

In an infected person, HIV persists as a chronic infection and in most cases AIDS ultimately develops, even in the presence of specific immune responses against the

21

virus. Thus, it is not completely clear what type of immune response(s) a vaccine should induce to protect against HIV/AIDS. In other words, we do not know what the 'immune correlates of protection' are.

Nevertheless, different types of experimental vaccines have been developed and some have been shown to induce various levels of protection in monkeys and chimpanzees challenged with virulent viruses. These animal protection experiments are perhaps the most compelling reason to believe that the development of an HIV vaccine is possible. However, we cannot be absolutely sure. We do not know what immune responses are protecting these animals, nor do we know what is the relevance of animal protection experiments in relation to potential vaccine-induced protection in humans.

Most vaccines against other viral infections are based on inactivated or attenuated (non-pathogenic) preparations of the virus. However, for safety reasons, these classical approaches for vaccine development are not being used for HIV/AIDS.

Instead, experimental (candidate) vaccines for HIV/AIDS are based on parts of the virus produced by different genetic engineering techniques, to ensure that vaccination will never result in HIV infection. The first generation of HIV vaccines was based on the envelope protein of the virus (gp120 or gp160) produced by genetic engineering. These proteins, and also synthetic peptides based on these proteins, are designed to induce neutralising antibodies against the virus, an immune response that some scientists believe could be sufficient to protect against HIV infection. Subsequently, other approaches for HIV vaccines have been developed, including the use of non-pathogenic viruses as vectors or carriers of HIV genes (such as vaccinia virus or related avian poxviruses). More recently, direct immunisation with DNA coding for the relevant HIV proteins is also being studied. Live-vectors and DNA immunisation can be optimised to induce neutralising antibodies, as well as cell-mediated immunity, a different type of immune response that some believe essential for protection against HIV/AIDS. Combinations of different vaccination approaches are also being explored.

The first human trial of an HIV vaccine was conducted in the USA in 1987. Since then, more than 6,000 healthy HIV-negative volunteers have participated in Phase I/II trials of more than 25 different candidate vaccines. These phase I/II trials are conducted in small numbers of volunteers (20–50 in Phase I trials, and 200–500 in Phase II trials), and they have shown that the vaccines were safe and that they induced different levels of immune responses against HIV (immunogenicity). These Phase I/II trials provided important information to improve the immunogenicity of subsequent generation of candidate vaccines. In order to assess the protective efficacy of a candidate vaccine it is necessary to conduct large-scale Phase III trials. These trials require the participation of several thousands of HIV-negative volunteers at higher risk of HIV infection, with one half receiving the candidate vaccine, and the other half receiving a control or placebo. Vaccine efficacy is assessed by comparing the number of HIV infections after an appropriate follow-up period. Phase III trials are scientifically, logistically and ethically very complex, but they are the only way of discovering if a candidate vaccine protects against HIV infection or AIDS.

The first Phase III trials started in 1998 in the USA and in 1999 in Thailand, using different versions of gp120 protein based on locally circulating strains of the virus (subtype B in the USA and BE in Thailand). Initial results from those Phase III trials, which will enrol a total of 8,000 volunteers, are expected by the end of 2001.

The second scientific challenge posed by HIV vaccine development is the genetic variability of HIV. Genetic analysis of HIV strains isolated in different parts of the world, especially of their envelope genes, have been used to classify HIV-1 into three 'groups' (M, O and N). The most prevalent one by far is group M. M-viruses are sub-classified into ten genetic subtypes (from A to J). Subtype B is the most prevalent in the Americas and in Western Europe, and it is the one being used for most HIV vaccine work. The most frequent subtype in the world is subtype C, which is responsible for more than 50 per cent of all HIV infections, especially in southern Africa, in the Horn of Africa and in India. The other two major subtypes in Africa are A and D. In Thailand and South East Asia, subtype E is the most prevalent. What is not clear at the present time, however, is if we will need vaccines against every HIV genetic subtype, or if we can develop broadly reactive vaccines. That is an issue of enormous importance for HIV vaccine research, and will be one for future vaccine use.

Multiple Vaccine Trials in Human Volunteers will be Needed

The most rational approach to accelerate the development of an urgently needed vaccine is to explore different vaccine concepts in parallel, including the simultaneous conduct of clinical (human) trials in industrialised and developing countries. These multiple trials are needed to assess the safety, immunogenicity and protective efficacy of different types of vaccines against different strains of HIV, and in different populations. Animal experiments suggest, for instance, that it might be more difficult to protect against parenteral inoculation (such as is the case with intravenous drug users) than against different types of sexual exposure. Likewise, genetic and nutritional factors could influence the immunogenicity of candidate vaccines.

Ultimately, the answer to the burning question on the relevance of the HIV genetic subtypes for vaccine-induced protection will come from Phase III trials conducted with subtype specific candidate vaccines in different countries.

Although most human trials of HIV candidate vaccines have been conducted in the USA and Europe, some trials have also been conducted in developing countries. To be more precise, 12 trials have been conducted in developing countries since 1993; eight of them in Thailand and the others in Brazil, China, Cuba and

Uganda (the only trial in Africa is a Phase I/II trial, and was initiated in February 1999). Other African countries planning to conduct Phase I/II trials in the near future are Kenya and South Africa; India is developing a comprehensive HIV vaccine development strategy.

In addition, a second Phase III trial, using a prime-boost combination of a live canarypox vector expressing HIV proteins followed by gp120, is being planned for conduct in the USA and in selected countries in the Caribbean and South America.

Why are Developing Countries Not More Involved?

Developing countries stand to benefit the most from an HIV vaccine. Why then, are developing countries not more actively involved in this global effort? Why are heavily affected countries not demanding an increase in the level of support for HIV vaccine development from the international community?

The response is complex. On one hand, HIV vaccine research is relatively under-funded, especially if compared with the severity of the epidemic. The total public/private expenditure on HIV vaccine research in 1999 was less than US$300 million, most of it provided by the National Institutes of Health of the USA, with a large proportion being used for basic research. In contrast, expenditure on AIDS drugs in the USA and Europe in 1999 was in the order of US$3 billion. The situation with HIV vaccines, especially for vaccines which could be appropriate for developing countries, can be qualified as a 'market failure', due to a combination of 'uncertain' scientific knowledge, difficulties in the conduct of trials in developing countries and lack of financial incentives to manufacturers.

On the other hand, developing countries may still have to understand the role that they must play if an HIV vaccine is ever going to be developed for those countries. And we must also understand their concerns:

- Heavily affected countries, especially in sub-Saharan Africa, are experiencing an ever-increasing number of AIDS cases, and they must provide care and treatment for those patients today. Under that pressure, only the most enlightened leaders would understand the importance of engaging on the long, uncertain and difficult road leading to the development of an HIV vaccine.

- The experience in most developing countries is that drugs and vaccines are developed in the 'North' and that they will eventually come to the 'South'. Given that perspective, developing countries may feel that they have no role to play in the process of HIV vaccine development. As discussed above, the genetic variability of HIV imposes the need to develop candidate vaccines based on strains prevalent in developing countries, and to conduct the appropriate human trials in these countries.

- There are many ethical and practical issues acting as disincentives for vaccine research in developing countries. The long-term nature of vaccine research requires commitment over a period of several years. That commitment will only come when national authorities and communities are satisfied that no ethical shortcuts will be taken in the conduct of the trials, and that the results of the research will benefit their populations. In this regard, UNAIDS recently released a guidance document on 'Ethical Considerations in HIV Preventive Vaccine Research', stressing the ethical responsibility of all sponsors of vaccine trials to make an effective vaccine available to all participants, as well as to other populations at high risk of HIV infection. Plans should be developed at the initial stages of HIV vaccine development to ensure such availability.

To ensure that a future HIV vaccine actually helps to control the HIV/AIDS pandemic, especially in developing countries, it is essential to start considering without delay how to organise and finance vaccine availability and delivery. This will require consultation and collaboration with communities, governments, donor agencies and the pharmaceutical industry, to ensure optimal coverage and sustainability. A minimum level of health services will also be required to enable appropriate programme implementation.

The Role of the World Health Organisation and UNAIDS

The development of an HIV vaccine will require the participation of multiple partners in the public and private sectors, in industrialised and developing countries, and this effort will have to be well co-ordinated in order to avoid unnecessary duplication and waste.

WHO has been actively involved in HIV vaccine activities since 1989. WHO and UNAIDS have now joined together to establish an HIV Vaccine Initiative, to take advantage of the comparative expertise of both organisations and to boost the international effort to develop appropriate HIV vaccines, with a special focus on developing countries. The new initiative will continue the activities of both organisations, focusing on:

- Advocacy, information and education – placing vaccines in the context of overall HIV prevention;

- Guidance and co-ordination of the international effort – developing norms and standards and acting as an 'honest broker' providing advice and support to developing countries considering the conduct of HIV vaccine trials. International co-ordination is provided through the WHO-UNAIDS 'Vaccine Advisory Committee';

- Promotion of appropriate vaccines for developing countries. Although not directly involved in product development, WHO-UNAIDS facilitates development of vaccines against strains prevalent in developing countries. This activity is co-ordinated by the WHO-UNAIDS Network for HIV Isolation and Characterisation;

- Facilitation of trials in developing countries – this is being done through targeted training, research and capacity building. These activities are implemented within the framework of WHO/UNAIDS-sponsored National AIDS Vaccine Plans (the first ones were developed in 1992–3 with Brazil, Thailand and Uganda). New strategies include the development of regional AIDS vaccine networks (the first one is being developed as part of a comprehensive 'African Strategy for AIDS Vaccines', a technical component of the International Partnership against AIDS in Africa);

- Planning future availability of HIV vaccines. When a safe and effective vaccine has been developed, this will become a major challenge for the international community.

Social Sectors – Meeting the Challenge

Religious Youth Groups Working Together

Andrew Hobbs and Richard Mambwe

'Consult and involve' were the principles guiding the development of a unique sexual health training manual for religious youth groups in Zambia, southern Africa. Young leaders of Christian and Muslim youth groups were at the centre of the process and are now training others on how to use their book, *Treasuring The Gift: How To Handle God's Gift Of Sex*. This participatory approach achieved the following:

- it helped religious leaders agree on how to help their young people avoid HIV;

- it resulted in a book that was highly relevant because it was produced by members of its target group;

- many different groups felt that this was their book, thereby increasing the chances of it being widely used; and

- it produced a team of able young peer educators.

Background

Zambia, in the centre of southern Africa, has one of the highest HIV rates in the world – 19 per cent of adults. The rate of new infections has peaked in the towns and cities, but is still rising in the countryside. Until recently Zambian society was rural and agrarian, with strong moral codes passed on and supported by extended families. People married young – marriage coming only a year or two after puberty.

Today, Zambia is the most urbanised country in Africa and neither tribal traditions nor Christianity nor Islam have caught up with the fact that marriage in modern Zambia now takes place many years after puberty. During this period before marriage, young people's hormones are telling them one thing, while religion and tradition tell them another.

Religious groups, particularly the Christian churches, have led the way in caring for individuals and families affected by AIDS, and in 1997 an inter-faith networking group, called Interfaith, was formed by Christians, Muslims and Bahai believers in Lusaka, with support from Robie Siamwiza, Technical Advisor for Policy with the organisation Project Concern International (PCI), an American charity. This group agreed to put aside differences in faith and doctrine in order to promote a united front against HIV/AIDS.

'The Lusaka Interfaith members are pretty progressive', says Karen Romano, Senior

Technical Adviser with PCI. 'They have taken on the challenge of working in HIV/AIDS prevention and have gone through much sensitisation and soul-searching, confronting the realities of people's lives.' This proved to be essential preparation for the group's support for the new training manual.

The Project

The Request

It was decided that what was needed was a participatory training resource for religious youth groups which did not require literacy.

Andrew Hobbs had previously worked with Karen Romano on the publication, *Happy, Healthy & Safe*, a peer education training manual for trainers as young as 14 years old. Karen Romano suggested that he should produce a second edition, containing activities requiring little or no literacy and targeted at religious youth groups. She observed:

It really struck me that the Church is the only pervasive, sustained network which brings not only youth but community members together, in every community in Zambia. No other organisation will ever compare in reach, and they are screaming for material to use in their HIV/AIDS outreach programmes.

Literature Search

In early 1998 a literature search, via electronic mailing lists and agencies in Britain and overseas, found few sexual health programmes aimed at religious youth groups. The exceptions were 'Scripture Union-Africa' and its series of 'Aid for AIDS' publications and the US charity organisation, 'Focus On The Family', whose videos and manuals promote sexual abstinence rather than the use of condoms. The latter's highly selective review of condom research is also used in a Ugandan manual, adapted by the Zambian Catholic Church, entitled *Behaviour Change Process*.

All these materials offer only the 'Plan A' of ideal sexual behaviour – no sex without marriage – without acknowledging that religions sometimes offer a 'Plan B' to reduce the harm or distress caused when people fail to live up to the ideal (divorce being one example). Our team was determined to incorporate into our project participatory learning methods such as role play, discussion, flow-charting and games, because of their suitability for exploring attitudes and practising skills.

Gaining Support from Religious Leaders

The next step was to win the trust of the Lusaka Interfaith HIV/AIDS networking group. Andrew was introduced by Robie Siamwiza, whose links with the group gave added instant credibility. It also helped that they had already identified a need for education materials for young people. Andrew met key members individually and in May 1998 Interfaith gave its full approval for the project.

Recruiting a Production Team

As a foreigner, Andrew needed some 'cultural interpreters' and in this he was ably assisted by Richard Mambwe, a talented young writer and researcher; Mary Simasiku of CARE-Zambia, an experienced user of Participatory Learning and Action (PLA) methods; and Holo Hachonda, who was knowledgeable about HIV prevention-training with religious youth groups.

Three women and seven men, aged 18–23 (two Muslim and eight Christian), were recruited, mainly from Interfaith members' youth clubs. Exceptionally talented and committed, they worked on the programme one or two days a week for expenses only – even during the World Cup! Andrew and Richard gained permission from the young people's religious leaders to pilot the learning activities in their churches and mosques. Such face-to-face advocacy and consultation paid dividends.

Training the Team

The project began with three days of training on sexual health and participatory methods, including a gender awareness session from a Zambian nun who runs a women's refuge. The team decided that the following topics should be covered:

- values
- recognising risk communication skills
- positive and negative peer pressure
- sexual relationships
- biological facts
- where to get help
- how to talk to parents
- how to live positively with HIV.

The Production Process: A Cycle of Action and Reflection

The whole team met every Thursday over a period of seven weeks. Andrew and Richard would draft instructions for two or three participatory learning activities; sometimes these were entirely their own creations and sometimes they adapted activities from other books (mainly from *Happy, Healthy & Safe*). During the meetings team members would lead an activity and afterwards the team reviewed the content and instructions and coached facilitation skills. The team aimed to make the Thursday meetings fun.

Each week team members introduced the activities rehearsed at the previous Thursday meeting to their local youth clubs. At the subsequent Thursday team meeting the members reported on how the activities had been received by the youth clubs, and improvements were then suggested and incorporated into each activity. Between team meetings, Andrew and Richard researched and wrote the background biology and theology for each activity, and Andrew re-drafted previous instructions.

Twice during this period the team met religious leaders from the Interfaith group and reviewed the project drafts together. Their response was encouraging. Robie Siamwiza commented, 'The opportunity for the various faiths to review the book and have input was very helpful. I think this helped to blunt any negative criticism.'

The Young People Start to Take Over!

As our weekly meetings hurtled by, something unexpected began to happen. Instead of the young people using the activities devised by Andrew and Richard, they began to devise their own. For example, they invented a scenario on how to talk to parents about boyfriends and girlfriends; they came up with two possibilities, which we reviewed together before choosing the best one.

This particular activity was a two-minute unfinished sketch concerning a mother who becomes outraged when her daughter asks a question about pregnancy. There were suggested discussion questions, a role play to practise broaching difficult subjects with parents and a final discussion. This exercise was as good as anything in a modern training manual.

The team members also developed into able and confident facilitators. They contributed to the background information, helped to brief an illustrator, planned (and appeared) in the book's photographs and chose the title. During the final meeting there was a discussion on how the book could best be disseminated – everyone in the team was impatient to get out there and show other young people their book.

The Finished Product

Two months after the Interfaith group gave the go-ahead, they were presented with a 142-page draft that contained 18 learning activities and was supported by 47 pages of background information.

Treasuring The Gift was launched at a national conference by a Zambian Government Minister, and it will form part of a life skills programme in schools. Robie Siamwiza says of the manual: 'UNICEF-Zambia are hailing it as a unique resource book for religious youth that actually discusses condom use!' Because of the popularity and acceptability of drama among Zambian young people, the manual relies heavily on drama, particularly unfinished sketches and role playing.

The manual has been disseminated through the churches and Islamic and Bahai groups involved in its production, and through the young people who helped to produce it. These young people played a key role in training and some of them have gone on to be recruited by their churches as peer educators.

Conclusion

Treasuring The Gift was fortunate in having all the ingredients for success:

- direct involvement of the target group, creating wide ownership of the process and the product;

- supportive commissioners who had thought through the issues and identified a need;

- adequate funding – the budget was £6,250 (sterling), funded by PCI;

- continuous consultation with all interested parties;

- a high level of motivation and ability in the production team.

Only time can tell if the book can contribute to the reduction of HIV infections in Zambia.

The following two pages are samples from *Treasuring The Gift: How To Handle God's Gift Of Sex*.

Topic 3 Communication skills

3c. Talking to parents

To help us talk to our parents more freely about relationships and sex

Read all of the exercise to make sure you understand everything

Practise translating the exercise into your local language

Read the NOTES FOR LEADERS

Choose 3 people to act the unfinished sketch, 'Talking To Parents'

Let the actors rehearse before the meeting so that they can do the sketch nicely

Watch unfinished sketch

Talk about the sketch

In two's, role-play child trying to talk to parent about a sensitive issue

Watch two of the role-plays

Talk about the role-plays

Introduction

First of all we are going to watch a short unfinished sketch.

What did you see in the sketch?

What subjects are difficult to talk about with parents?

Why is it taboo to talk about such subjects with parents?

What can be done to help parents and children talk about such issues?

Does anyone have any techniques or strategies for talking about difficult subjects with their parents? Can you share with us the ways you use?

Now let us get into pairs (two by two) and do a short role-play.

One person is a parent, the other is a child. The child should try to discuss a difficult subject with the parent.

Give 5 minutes.

You should go round and watch the role-plays, to see which is a good example of an understanding parent, and which is a good example of a parent who refuses to discuss such subjects.

Unfinished Sketch

Talking To Parents

A girl asks her mother: Is it true that a girl cannot get pregnant, the first time she has sex?

The mother is shocked, and tells her daughter she should be ashamed, to mention such things to her mother. It is taboo.

At this point the brother comes in, and agrees with his sister: the youth need to know these things, and it is better to learn them from our parents.

The mother says that they should ask their grandmother such questions, not their mother.

'But our grandmother stays far away,' the sister and brother reply.

[The actors freeze at this point.]

A Church Perspective

Catholic Agency for Overseas Development (CAFOD)

What are the HIV/AIDS Issues for Faith Communities?

The particular faith community within which we locate this question is that of the Catholic Church. The social teachings of the Catholic Church underpin the essential link between faith and justice and stress the unique value of each human being and the rights of all to share in the resources at our disposal. These teachings articulate our responsibility to establish and uphold conditions that bring justice and equity and in this regard to side preferentially with the poorest and least powerful.

This body of teaching charges our faith community to respond with unreserved solidarity and compassion (in the truest sense of this word) to people infected or affected by HIV and to tackle the many and diverse issues of institutional and personal injustice highlighted by the HIV/AIDS pandemic. It is within this framework that the issues described below and the challenges they pose are set.

HIV is a Development Issue

While recognising the important health concern that HIV is for those infected, the disproportionate impact of HIV/AIDS on third world countries makes it a development issue requiring urgent attention. An estimated 95 per cent of people with HIV or AIDS live in developing countries. In some of these countries 10–25 per cent of the adult population is infected. The effects on communities and countries are devastating.

The majority of adults with HIV are in the 25–49 age group. The consequences for local and national economies are stark, in both the agricultural and industrial sectors, because of hugely reduced productivity and absenteeism due to sickness, care requirements of other sick family members and attendance at funerals. Additionally, skills lost to industry, agriculture, education, health care and other essential areas cannot be easily or quickly replaced. As well as the immediate and longer-term repercussions of this on communities' well-being and prosperity, it also deprives future generations of educational and training opportunities.

The health gains of the last 30 years in many countries have already been reversed because of HIV/AIDS. Life expectancy in the countries of southern Africa had risen from 44 years in the early 1950s to 59 years in the early 1990s. Because of HIV/AIDS it is set to recede to 45 years between 2005 and 2010, its lowest level in half a century. Child mortality rates are similarly affected, with the reductions of the early 1980s being followed by a significant upturn by the end of that decade in countries of Africa where HIV prevalence was highest. Although the epidemic is younger in Asian countries, it is anticipated that here too similar reversals will emerge.

The loss of a considerable proportion of the adult population is also leaving large numbers of orphaned children. The traditional caring system of the extended family is no longer able to cope in many parts of Africa and many of these children end up surviving by whatever means on the streets of towns and larger cities. As well as the effects of this on their physical and emotional well-being, these children are often vulnerable to sexual exploitation and HIV infection. Grandparents who rely on their adult children to care for them in their old age are robbed of this security and instead carry the extra burden of trying to care for their orphaned grandchildren.

Poverty and Inequality of Resources

Although 95 per cent of people with HIV/AIDS are in developing countries, less than 10 per cent of the total expenditure on HIV prevention or care is spent in these countries.

Poverty goes hand in hand with HIV/AIDS. Poverty increases people's vulnerability to HIV infection on many counts. Lack of access to education reduces people's capacity for economic survival and also makes them less likely to access education about HIV and wider sexual health education. Similarly, inability to access general health care and early treatment for other sexually transmitted diseases increases vulnerability to HIV. Inability to access voluntary HIV testing also needs to be named in this context. Less than one in ten people worldwide know they have HIV and thus cannot take this into considerations about sexual behaviour, reproductive choices, etc. Absence of alternative sources of income drives many women and young girls (and increasingly young boys) to barter their only commodity, sex, for food, school fees or other essentials for themselves or their families.

HIV also plunges families into poverty. Family income drops as wage earners become sick or fields are left untended. Remaining resources are often spent on medical care, children (usually girls) are taken out of school to care for ailing parents or because they cannot pay school fees.

Inequality of resources at international level means that the antiretrovirals so valuable in the North in improving the health of people with HIV or preventing mother-to-child transmission of the virus are beyond the reach of all but the very rich in developing countries. Additionally, even inexpensive drugs to alleviate pain or treat typical HIV-related infections like TB or thrush are unavailable in many parts.

The burden of debt and of structural adjustment programmes and similar measures imposed by the North exacerbates the intolerable situation of most people worldwide infected by HIV and increases the vulnerability of those not infected. The implication of unjustified levels of profit pursued by pharmaceutical companies along with corruption, ineptitude or lack of accountability within governments of some countries of the South needs also to be acknowledged.

Power Imbalances

Circumstances that augment imbalances of power between individuals and between groups increase the spread of HIV infection. In all countries of the world, power imbalances occur between the prosperous and the poor, between men and women, between people who know they are infected by HIV and those who believe themselves not to be infected, and between adults and children. Power imbalances also occur against groups already marginalised, for example because of sexual orientation, ethnicity and lifestyles such as drug use that are deemed anti-social. Such imbalances are often reinforced by culture, politics, legislation, religion, economic policies and social expectations.

Challenges to the Beliefs of Faith Communities

HIV has highlighted the ongoing struggles of Church and other faith communities with their understanding of sexuality with regard to behaviour and orientation. It has also highlighted the positive contribution that faith communities can make to a wider understanding of sexuality that affirms the unique yet equal value and dignity of each human being.

HIV has also exposed the injustices committed by Church and other faith communities that promulgate an image of a wrathful God: communities that judge, exclude, stigmatise and otherwise discriminate against those who do not or cannot conform, or those who, simply, are different. It has called for prophetic voices to name the injustices highlighted by HIV, whether they occur within these communities or more widely at community, economic, social and political levels nationally and internationally.

How does the Catholic Faith Community Respond to the Issues?

It is impossible to give a complete account of the Catholic community's response, varying as it does in the very different cultural and economic contexts of countries North and South. The following is written from CAFOD's experience as the development agency of the Catholic Church of England and Wales supporting partners in Africa, Asia, Latin America and Eastern Europe. From this perspective we can say that the Catholic faith community responds in two directions.

The first direction is that of the many and varied responses by local faith-based community programmes. The Catholic Church (and other Christian churches) particularly in many parts of Africa and to a lesser degree in Latin America, has structures in place that deliver health care, education and social welfare provision. It also has vibrant community groups and many skilled and experienced community-based organisations, all of which are natural channels for a concerted response to HIV and AIDS. Programmes developed within these channels have included home-based and community-based care initiatives for people with AIDS, counselling and pastoral care, projects to care for orphans and vulnerable children, to provide voluntary HIV testing and counselling, to enable income generation schemes, HIV education and prevention initiatives, peer education projects, youth work, women's empowerment, lobbying and advocacy work, and much more. Often communities integrate HIV-related considerations into pre-existing initiatives and structures; in other instances they develop new approaches and projects to specifically address the concerns posed by HIV.

CAFOD is the lead agency for HIV/AIDS within Caritas which is the worldwide confederation of Catholic emergency, relief and development agencies. It is at this level that the second direction of response of the Catholic faith community finds expression. CAFOD works though this confederation to enable HIV/AIDS to be an integral part of church-based programmes by opening up debate with bishops' conferences at national and regional levels mainly, though not entirely, in countries of the South. In this capacity CAFOD offers workshops, seminars and fora for theological debate to enable bishops to consider HIV as a complex issue with pastoral, theological, economic, gender-related, social, health and human rights implications which the Church cannot turn its back on. Similar initiatives have been undertaken with priests and male and female religious communities. This work with bishops, priests and members of religious communities is in recognition of their important roles as gatekeepers of the communities within their area of influence. Gaining the support and commitment of these gatekeepers is an essential first step. Lack of such commitment can either block the possibility of any response at programmatic level or allow communities to continue in the seemingly more comfortable option of denial or silence. At its worst it can generate a response that stigmatises, excludes and judges.

The response of the Catholic faith community can never be formulated in isolation. HIV-related issues need to be part of the Church's wider endeavours to enhance justice, human rights and development. Church-based responses likewise need to form part of the wider community, governmental (as appropriate to local context) and international HIV-related initiatives. One expression of the latter is the Memorandum of Understanding drawn up in 1998 between Caritas and UNAIDS, pledging a collaborative response to the challenges of HIV/AIDS, with each organisation contributing its strengths and particular expertise while respecting differences of approach and understanding where these legitimately exist.

Suggestions for Commonwealth Collaborative Action across the Sectors

Commonwealth organisations can show a commonality and empathy with the human rights, justice and development issues that evoke a response to HIV/AIDS from faith communities by:

• Identifying opportunities within each sector to address the inter-relationship between HIV and the development and human rights issues referred to here;

• Engaging in campaigns at national and international level that advocate for greater equality in distribution of resources and seek to ease debt burdens that hamper efforts to assuage the impact of HIV;

• Lobbying for a sustained commitment from national governments, South and North, and international agencies such as the UN, World Bank, etc to providing longer-term effective responses and not just politically motivated 'quick fixes';

• Mobilising all relevant players within a country – communities, business sector, faith groups, governments and voluntary organisations to provide a concerted response to HIV prevention and support needs. This includes actively involving people living with HIV in planning and implementing, as individual skills and capacities allow;

• Recognising the indispensable roles of faith communities in any effort to prevent HIV infection and provide support for people already infected. This requires that Commonwealth organisations recognise and incorporate the strengths of faith communities while working within the limitations of their agreed boundaries. It also requires that the sectors acknowledge that they can learn from and contribute to the role played by faith communities confronting the challenges posed by HIV/AIDS.

Acknowledgement

This material was originally presented at the conference 'The HIV/AIDS Crisis: A Commonwealth Response', Marlborough House, London, 7 December 2000.

HIV/AIDS and Religion: Exploring Pathways for Local Community and Political Response

Ian D Campbell

Religion is a structural representation of personal faith within people. This current of faith is often neglected in deference to debate about religious organisations and leadership.

The primary health care movement of the 1970s revolutionised patterns of health promotion and care. Yet HIV/AIDS impact in families, neighbourhoods and countries has challenged health and development workers to look again at the concept and practice, and at other approaches to nurturing local community involvement. People often feel defeated, especially in high prevalence situations, because the usual approaches are not working.

Why is this so? Is it connected to the fact that HIV is transmitted sexually and through infected blood? Is it that there is linkage between sexuality, relationships, intimacy and behaviours, which standard health approaches do not address? Exploration and expression of this link is strongly influenced by culture and by religious faith. Health and development interventions do not always respect this influence, yet should do so if the capacity for a truly passionate response in people is to be developed.

Whilst spirituality and faith are elements of local community capacity that are not often especially acknowledged, spiritual health is the ultimate intimacy. People in religious organisations need therefore to be recognised as key participants in local and national responses. For example, the Churches Medical Association of Zambia represents 50 per cent of rural health work in the country, and 30 per cent nationally. Yet so often they are on the margins in the minds of donors and government, whilst frequently contributing enormously to national response.

Primary Health Care

We need to reflect carefully on this lack of acknowledgement of spiritual life, especially in primary health care work. Decentralised health services are not the essence of primary health care. Community participation and ownership of responsibility are central principles. Yet in the often painful process of organisational development, hospitals and health departments have not really been a source of genuine facilitation, which means letting go of power and helping local communities to succeed. Primary health care as it is often practised can touch local communities, yet does not go far enough. It organises, it creates access, it trains, yet does it enter authentically into the aura of community belonging based in 'everyday' relatedness of families and neighbourhoods? Does it cultivate this kind of community building when the relatedness is fractured?

It may do so if those involved really believe in the capacity of the local community – yet so often it does not, because the implementers do not facilitate expansion of capacity. They retain power and do not really participate; they are self-focused rather than team-minded.

In responding to HIV/AIDS much more is demanded of people. HIV is insidious. It has raged unchecked in locations where health work is excellent. Its genesis is based in a search for relationship by people trying to belong. They make choices and in participating in a response to HIV, local people need to feel they are developing by choice. They need confidence rather than fear, they need accompaniment rather than instruction. If this happens, then the way is open for solutions to many other health problems that communities confront.

A Movement toward Spiritual Health

It has only been in the last five years that more widespread recognition of local community relational and spiritual capacity has been shown by United Nations organisations and governments. Three examples at the international level are the African mayors' initiative of the United Nations Development Programme (HIV and Development,[1] New York); UNAIDS (Geneva) Local Response Team;[2] and the Washington-based NGO Health Networks workshop on shared confidentiality of February 2000, facilitated by the Salvation Army international headquarters programme facilitation team.[3]

Even prior to 1995 a theme consistently explored by some faith-based NGOs and churches has been the link of care to change, and therefore to prevention.[4] The context for this analysis has been home care by a team and its relationship to neighbourhood conversation, characterised by a counselling approach.

One major reflection to emerge has been expansion of the meanings contained in community health, to include a spectrum of sexual, reproductive, family and relational health. The journey toward explicit acknowledgement of spiritual capacity as part of the definition of health has started and the impact of HIV/AIDS is a major contributor.

This acknowledgement is critical to effective community response. Intimate sexual and drug using behaviours do not change easily, yet faith-based motivation is a hugely powerful internal response that is largely untapped. Politics, environment, poverty, gender insensitivity and power inequity influence motivation but do not touch the soul of a community in the same way as relationship-based respect for spiritual capacity. Facilitation of local family and neighbourhood spiritual connectedness is a key foundation for effective response.

But how can a health team enter the heartbeat, the soul and spirit of a community? Clearly, by invitation, with appreciation of local strengths and a belief in the capacity of local people to care, belong, change and hope. Yet also with an almost mystical and sometimes explicit acknowledgement of spiritual capacity inevitably linked to belonging to the future as well as the past and present. This approach generates hope for quality of life, and allows for adequate remembering and continuity even with the reality of accumulating loss.

Religion and HIV/AIDS

The connection of HIV/AIDS and a national response to religion is best developed within a recognition of local spiritual capacity. The framework for engagement between religion and HIV/AIDS is broader, encompassing not only the essential faith of people but also religious leadership and religious organisations.

This distinction is key to engaging the strength of religious movements and organisations. So often religious organisations and leaders have obstructed response. Often this has happened in a context of passionate defence by religious leadership of moral principle, entirely consistent with their vocation and vision of service to God and to people; yet also with too much distance from local reality.

As leaders engage in the life situation of people with HIV, almost inevitably their perspective shifts. This was the case for those involved in exposure visits preceding the consultation of church leaders with UNAIDS held in Botswana in September 1999.[5] As leaders met with families with AIDS/HIV in their homes, and as they participated in neighbourhood discussions, pain was felt, compassion deepened and commitment to involvement grew.

There are other examples of innovative engagement, through which some pathways for shared response can develop – including religious organisations and faith-motivated neighbourhoods and other communities, within wider societal and political response.

The Botswana consultation was part of an African initiative to strengthen action by people of Christian faith in their own local communities, as part of those communities, and also as part of the church.

Examples already exist, and are developing, of interfaith dialogue and co-operation in relation to HIV/AIDS. These include:

- The Conference on AIDS and Religion held in Senegal in 1998.[6] After a presentation by a Christian organisation of community- and home-based approaches within countries such as India, Haiti, Kenya and the Philippines, an Imam commented: 'We can work together in the community. We believe in family and reconciliation with God. You believe in relationship between people representing the process of relationship to God. Government is promoting community ownership which depends on good relationship. We can all share on this point.'

- An initiative in Hikkadua town, south of Colombo, Sri Lanka, where a Christian team which has been doing home visits in Buddhist neighbourhoods for four years has recently been invited to the local Buddhist temple to facilitate discussion between attenders from the local community.[7]

- The Africa Regional Forum of Religious Health Organisations in Reproductive Health, based on a partnership between religious health networks, Christian and Islamic. The Forum, facilitated by International Family Health, was launched at the International Conference on AIDS and STDs in Africa, September 1999.[8]

- A series of meetings sponsored by the UK NGO, AIDS Consortium, on responses to HIV/AIDS by faith-based organisations.[9]

- The draft declaration of UNGASS (April 2001) which affirms the necessity of faith-based organisational response.[10]

These and other examples represent increased confidence within secular organisations to explicitly affirm, respect and engage with religious organisations and faith-based communities.

What are we Learning?
Some Collaborative Pathways

None of us is strong enough to achieve alone all that is needed. We know that we cannot often do the same work because we have different strengths, yet we can strengthen each other through sharing our vision about care, change, the potential for community as healthy belonging and about hope. Another pathway is commitment to participatory ways of working, thinking and being. Another is commitment to shared desirable outcomes, especially those associated with community capacity development.

Some Distinctions

There is a difference in context between religious organisations, religious leadership and personal faith. All are valued facets of religious identity, yet the fact that most people hold some form of personal, spiritual faith is too rarely acknowledged within international policy that is concerned with societal response. Why is this so? Is it that personal spiritual faith is the ultimate intimacy? Has spirituality been left out of the term 'holistic health'?

'Morality' can be received as affirmation of the mutual good, without assumption or judgement or exclusion. It can be an expression of solidarity, including beliefs that are offered and often owned by the wider community. Articulation of religious values and norms can be part of the community identity rather than an imposition.

There can be dysfunction between beliefs and practice in any organisation. With religious leaders, vision is not generally in question, because it is not difficult for people to easily subscribe to the concepts of loving care and the need for hope. However, corresponding practices are often in question. For example, instead of a participatory approach, an imposing or provider approach is dominant. For the religious sector, there is an immediate need to develop convictional motivation based on theological grounding for both beliefs and practices (see Vision and Direction Framework developed for the Consultation with Christian Leaders, Development Organisations and UNAIDS on HIV/AIDS Related Issues, held in Botswana in September 1999).

Distinction between Public Disclosure and Shared Confidentiality
Shared confidentiality is shared knowledge and understanding of meanings within a context of respectful intimacy within a group in which there is a sense of mutual accountability. Knowledge that is shared in this context is not a secret. The content and meanings are known within the group, even though there is not necessarily open conversation about the content and meanings. It is possible to counsel a community on the basis of shared confidentiality, without HIV-positive members of the group having to verbally disclose their status, and this has been found to be an effective environment for stigma reduction and normalisation.

Key relevant themes drawn from local community capacity development approaches relevant to destigmatisation:

* Care

  A supportive presence that accompanies people in their situation, for example, visiting a neighbour or a community visit. Care reflects mutual support between family, neighbours, community, and a relationship of being with, and interacting with, others.

* Change

  Change occurs by seeing care (or experiencing care), which leads people to acknowledge the reality of HIV, and may result in a change in understanding and attitude. Care helps to make change more likely to happen. Change does not happen simply in people in isolation but when the care and change process is relational in nature, change is expansive. It is a foundation for going to scale.

Link between Care and Change
The link between care and change is relational. Care that is personal and is observed by people in the household and neighbourhood can generate motivation and action for shared change. This can rapidly shift a situation from stigma to shared responsibility for change around issues of mutual concern.

The care to change linkage is also termed 'care/prevention' linkage. It is a key strategic approach to expansion of circles of involvement in local community and organisational responses to HIV/AIDS.

There is an emerging maturity of expression and action within secular and religious organisations. Politicians can do more to affirm the power of spiritual belief, and to understand the core vision of religious leaders and the values within religious movements. Yet 'religion' can and should more actively accompany the pain of accumulating loss in local communities and be part of shared growth in faith and hope.

Notes

1. Available from United Nations Development Programme (HIV and Development Programme, New York), 304 East 45th Street, New York, NY 10017, USA. E-mail: mina.mauerstein-bail@undp.org

2. UNAIDS (Geneva). Keynotes 1 and 2 (drafts) of the Local Response Team, March 2000. E-mail: unaids@unaids.org. www.unaids.org

3. Available from NGO Health Networks workshop on shared confidentiality, February 2000. Networks for Health, 1620 1 Street NW, Suite 900, Washington DC 20006, USA. E-mail: rhope@dc.savechildren.org

4. Campbell, I and Rader, A (1995). 'HIV counselling in developing countries: the link from individual to community counselling for support and change', British Journal of Guidance and Counselling, Vol 23: No. 1.

5. Consultation with Christian Development Organisations and UNAIDS for Collaboration on HIV/AIDS-Related Issues, Botswana (March 2000), Journey into Hope.

6. First International Conference on AIDS and Religion, Dakar, Senegal (1997), sponsored by UNAIDS, Geneva. www.unaids.org

7. Report of the first cross-regional consultation of programme facilitation teams (India and Asia/Pacific). February 2000. The Salvation Army International Headquarters, London, UK.

8. Xth International Conference on AIDS and STDs in Africa, 12–16 September 1999, Lusaka, Zambia, African Regional Forum of Religious Health Organisations in Reproductive Health – an initiative to promote opportunities for increased advocacy and experience sharing among religious health organisations in Africa, prepared by International Family Health, Parchment House, 13 Northburgh Street, London EC1V OJP.

9. UK NGO AIDS Consortium. February 2000. E-mail: ukaidscon@gn.apc.org

10. Available through the UNAIDS, www.unaids.org

A Trade Union Perspective

Annie Watson

Introduction

The Commonwealth Trade Union Council is composed of the trade union national centres, representing 30 million trade union members, throughout the Commonwealth. We recognised many years ago that we have an important role to play in the fight against HIV/AIDS and our member organisations have been actively promoting policies to address the issue. We welcome the concern expressed by Commonwealth Heads of Government in Paragraph 55 of the communiqué summarising the conclusions of the 1999 Durban Commonwealth Heads of Government Meeting.

Trade unionists campaign to uphold the values which unite them, regardless of the level of economic development of any country. These values of non-discrimination, protection of children and vulnerable groups, gender equality, public service efficiency and government accountability are all challenged by the impact of HIV/AIDS.

HIV/AIDS Issues in the Trade Union Sector

Thousands of workers are victimised because of pre-employment mandatory testing; their suffering remains hidden because of the atmosphere of fear and shame surrounding HIV status. Those in work experience discrimination when their HIV status becomes known. They are likely to face unfair dismissal, harassment, lack of confidentiality and denial of promotion. Denial of vocational training is a recurring abuse faced by HIV-positive workers because employers do not want to invest in people they expect will be sick. HIV-positive workers also face discrimination by their fellow workers. Sometimes they refuse to work with them, insist that they take breaks away from other workers and that they eat alone. In many countries there are cultural barriers to open discussion about sexual practices which make workplace education difficult to implement.

Some workers are exposed to risk of HIV infection, through contact with infected blood or body fluids in the course of their work. These include health care workers, police officers, emergency service workers, prison workers, teachers and hotel workers. Other categories of workers who spend long periods away from home are also vulnerable to infection. Many workers in mining, transport and fishing see their families only twice a year and are likely to have multiple and casual sexual relationships, increasing the risk of HIV infection.

Workers in the informal sector account for a large section of the workforce in developing countries. Due to the lack of regulation and monitoring of the informal sector, workers have few rights, little training and often work in unhealthy and unsafe conditions. In the vast majority of cases, they do not have access to information vital to prevent infection and are unable to exercise their right to protection against discrimination if infected. Workers with HIV/AIDS are forced to take on any work in order to survive, making them particularly vulnerable to exploitation.

The gender dimension to poverty and inequality helps to explain women's greater vulnerability to HIV infection. Inequality in employment and wages reinforces women's financial dependency on men and reduces a woman's power to insist on safer sexual practices. The need to supplement income results in many women selling sex either as prostitutes or in less formal relationships. When the main breadwinner is no longer able to work, other family members, including children, are forced to work to supplement the family income. The number of children engaged in income-earning activities in countries with a high prevalence of HIV/AIDS increases significantly.

Trade unionists see that poverty aggravates the situation and creates favourable conditions for HIV/AIDS to spread. The increased number of people in need of medical attention because of HIV/AIDS stretches health care systems to breaking point. There is a lack of access to affordable drugs in many developing countries. In many Commonwealth countries, governments have not come to terms with the need to acknowledge the problem of HIV/AIDS and there is no national strategy to tackle it.

How Trade Unions are Addressing these Issues

Trade unionists in the Commonwealth are addressing the issues in several ways: through membership education programmes, through negotiation with employers and through national lobbying.

Membership Education Programmes

Trade union organisations in many Commonwealth countries have taken initiatives to distribute information to their members and other workers on prevention, treatment and care in relation to HIV/AIDS and on how to assist HIV-positive people. In South Africa, the national trade union federation, COSATU, has produced a handbook for shop stewards which explains that their role is to promote safe working practices, to protect workers with HIV/AIDS from discrimination and to support families when breadwinners are unable to work. In Uganda, the CTUC assisted the National Organisation of Trade Unions to develop a training manual for union educators to help spread awareness among union members. In Tanzania, the trade union federation has organised drama performances in workplaces and residential areas to promote awareness. In Kiribati, HIV/AIDS awareness has been included in the programme of First Aid training carried out by the Red Cross for all seafarers; trade union educators have noted a high level of understanding by their members as a result

Negotiation with Employers

There is great potential for joint employer/union co-operation to develop a comprehensive HIV/AIDS workplace policy and programme. A practical example of this is the 1991 AIDS Agreement between the National Union of Mineworkers and the Chamber of Mines in South Africa. The Agreement covers protection against discrimination, harassment and non-consensual testing, counselling, benefits, awareness and education programmes, and a ban on adverse employment consequences, including dismissal because of HIV infection. There is a similar agreement between trade unions in South Africa and the Ford Motor Company. In Zambia, there is a joint workplace education programme organised between the union and Barclays Bank. In Kiribati, the Overseas Seamen's Union campaigned to stop mandatory testing and to persuade employers not to terminate the employment of HIV-positive seafarers. In Tanzania, trade unionists have also been involved in a joint programme with employers to distribute condoms in the workplace.

National Lobbying

Trade unions are an important component of civil society lobbying activities on national issues. In South Africa, COSATU is part of the Treatment Action Campaign which emphasises the need for accessible primary health care, cheap drugs and to make life better for people living with HIV/AIDS. In many Commonwealth countries, trade unions are part of national debt networks which campaign for cancellation of the external debt of developing countries to enable increased expenditure on health and education programmes. Trade unionists point out that poor living conditions and low wages are factors which make it difficult for many people to change behaviour that puts them at risk of HIV infection.

Trade unionists also campaign to change public attitudes in those countries where there is a tendency to deny the existence of social problems. These can include alcoholism, child abuse, domestic violence, unwanted pregnancies and homophobia, as well as HIV/AIDS, and until the denial of the problem by the authorities is overcome there can be no progress in tackling it. In this area, alliances between trade unionists and other civil society organisations play an important part. Where governments have established task forces on HIV/AIDS, and have involved trade unionists as partners, they have played an important role. In Kiribati, a trade union leader chairs the government HIV/AIDS Task Force.

Suggestions for Commonwealth Collaborative Action

Action in the Trade Union Sector

Within the Commonwealth, much of the pioneering work in the trade union movement has taken place in South Africa, in a few other African countries and in some particular sectors, such as with transport workers. Trade unions have the potential to work in this way in every Commonwealth country, but education programmes are needed to raise awareness and to help trade unionists everywhere to learn from the experience in other countries. The CTUC will continue to support our sisters and brothers in the developing countries of the Commonwealth and to try to secure the resources for this work.

Action across Sectors

Workplace HIV/AIDS programmes are an important element in any HIV/AIDS strategy and serve to strengthen legislation at national level. These should be developed in partnership with trade unions at enterprise level and include the following elements:

- Prohibition on direct and indirect discrimination on the basis of HIV status;

- Protection of occupational benefits;

- Working time and conditions of employment should be adapted to facilitate necessary medical treatment;

- Education and information campaigns to prevent the spread of HIV/AIDS, addressing issues such as stigmatisation and encouraging a culture of openness;

- Strengthening occupational health and safety programmes to protect groups of workers who are particularly at risk;

- Free distribution and availability of condoms through the workplace;

- Protection of the right of privacy and confidentiality about the health status of workers;

- Free testing and counselling services.

We would like other agencies to see the potential in involving trade unions as partners.

For example, there could be a Commonwealth-wide campaign for joint union/ employer activities in every workplace on International Aids Day in 2001. We would like every Commonwealth government to establish a task force on HIV/ AIDS and to invite trade unions to be involved. In every aspect of this issue, it is important that examples of good practice are disseminated and replicated and the Commonwealth can help to make sure this happens. Trade unionists have a good record in campaigning for social justice and can make a big contribution to the fight against HIV/AIDS – we want to be involved.

Acknowledgement

This material was originally presented at the conference, 'The HIV/AIDS Crisis: A Commonwealth Response', Marlborough House, London, 7 December 2000.

HIV, Gender and Health

Clement Chela

HIV/AIDS – A Challenge of Global Proportions

Acquired Immune Deficiency Syndrome (AIDS), the disease caused by the Human Immuno-Deficiency Virus (HIV), was first recognised in the early 1980s. Initially the major routes of infection were through the sharing of needles among intravenous drug users and homosexual contacts. However, the main mode of spread is now through heterosexual intercourse, unsafe blood transfusions and maternal transmission to offspring in the perinatal period and through breastfeeding.

The scale of the HIV/AIDS epidemic has been increasing enormously from year to year and it has now grown to the proportions of a worldwide pandemic. It has already reached catastrophic proportions in a number of countries – particularly in Africa and Asia. At the present time, some 16 million people have already died since the start of the epidemic and around 33 million are known to be infected, 23 million of them in Africa. Infection rates in the adult population (15–49 years old) are typically in the range 20–26 per cent in a number of east, central and southern African countries.

Global HIV/AIDS Trends

The table below shows the global trends in HIV/AIDS since 1996 based on data collected by WHO and published in 1999.

The general trend is an increase in the number of men and women affected since 1996. However, recent studies have shown a decline in the prevalence of HIV in young people as a result of targeted campaigns among young men and women in Uganda and young male army conscripts in Thailand. This suggests some success in stemming the spread of the disease; however this is not so in surrounding countries where the epidemic continues to spread.

Impact of HIV on the Community

The epidemic has had, and continues to have, a detrimental impact on all aspects of community life. The long time lag between HIV infection, AIDS and death – more than 10 years on average – helps to explain why most countries have yet to see the damage the epidemic can do to their social and economic fabric. So far, the greatest impact is visible in sub-Saharan Africa, where the epidemic began in the late 1970s and has reached high levels of intensity. In this region, reports show that the epidemic is eclipsing health and other development gains that governments, citizens and development agencies have worked so hard to achieve.

Global Trends in HIV/AIDS, 1996–99

		1999	1996
People newly infected with HIV	Total	5,600,000	3,100,000
	Adults	5,000,000	2,700,000
	Women	*2,300,000*	—
	Children <15 years	570,000	400,000
People living with HIV/AIDS	Total	33,600,000	22,600,000
	Adults	32,4 00,000	21,800,000
	Women	*14,800,000*	*9,200,000*
	Children <15 years	1,200,000	830 000
AIDS deaths	Total	2,600,000	1,500,000
	Adults	2,100,000	1,100,000
	Women	*1,100,000*	*470 000*
	Children <15 years	470,000	350,000
Total AIDS deaths since the beginning of the epidemic	Total	16,300,000	6,400,000
	Adults	12,700,000	5,000,000
	Women	*6,200,000*	*2,100,000*
	Children <15 years	3,600,000	1,400,000

Impact on the Health Care System

The epidemic has had a profound impact on health services in most of the affected countries. Bed occupancy has reached levels of 60–85 per cent. This has exacerbated chronic shortages of equipment, supplies and medicines, making it more difficult to provide basic health services. Illness and absenteeism of health staff has also had a major impact on health services. The cost to the family is overwhelming with the ever-increasing cost of care through formal and traditional health systems. Despite these difficulties in the health care system, some useful responses, such as home care that involves the participation of communities and the family, have developed.

Treatments for controlling HIV, such as triple, double or combination antiretroviral therapy, have come into widespread use in the developed world over the past two years. Yet, because of cost (£10,000 per year) and difficulty of administration, they remain inaccessible to most people living with HIV in developing countries. Possible cost reductions using combinations of anti-viral and anti-cancer agents may help to increase access. Studies are still being evaluated on the benefits and possible ways these and other antiretroviral drugs can be made available in countries where the health budget is often insufficient to meet basic health needs. Recent studies have shown that a single dose of the antiretroviral, Nevirapine, given to an infected woman in labour, together with a dose given to her baby within three days of birth, halves the HIV transmission rate. This would potentially prevent some 300,000 to 400,000 babies per year from being born HIV-positive.

Impact on Households

The cost of care of the HIV-infected individual results in increased household spending to sustain their health. This leads to progressive impoverishment of families as the illness progresses. The loss of earnings through the illness of the breadwinner causes a further reduction in the household income. This rises dramatically with the death of the individual as the income is severed and followed by the additional expense of funeral and burial arrangements. In some instances the burden on the household is further increased by the loss of property to relatives through inheritance.

In the majority of cases the primary care givers are women who are expected to provide care in addition to the other work they do in the home. In many situations, for example where women also carry the burden of farming, this has been shown to reduce farm output for family consumption and sale. This further erodes the family's capacity to provide education and other services for their children.

In cases where both parents have died from AIDS, children are left to be cared for in orphanages or by the extended family system. Where these systems are non-existent the children are left in the care of their grandparents. This places an added burden on upon the grandparents, as they are less able to care for themselves and the orphans due to old age. In some severe cases children have been left on their own to fend for themselves. The eldest of the children often give up their education to provide necessary support for the younger siblings.

Where one or both parents are infected, their painful progression through the various stages from well-being to ill health and death, are constantly before the family members. This has been observed to have long-term psychological and emotional effects on children.

Impact on the Economy

AIDS affects individuals in their most productive years and leads to poor economic performance. These impacts begin to arise when the infected individual develops symptomatic HIV infection. This can result in the loss of productive work through absences and increased expenditure on medical and sick benefits. The impacts are particularly severe when there are few trained individuals to carry on the work of sick workers. Their replacement with junior and inexperienced staff can lead to poor decisions or damage to equipment. This has several consequences including reduced savings, reinvestment or spending and finally a downturn in the development of social and economic sectors.

Preventing new infections is ultimately the best way of preventing all these impacts. Success hinges on using a careful mix of tried-and-tested prevention methods. However, some of them, like sexual health education at school, or harm-reduction programmes for drug users, may be more costly in terms of political capital than the resources required for implementation.

AIDS and Gender

HIV/AIDS affects both women and men. To date, the majority of those who have been infected and those who have died have been men, but infection rates for women have risen steeply in the last few years. Gender analysis is crucial to understanding HIV/AIDS transmission. It highlights the socially constructed aspects of male-female relations that underpin individual behaviour, as well as the gender-based rules, norms and laws governing the broader social and institutional context. A correct analysis forms the basis for the changes required to create an environment in which men and women can protect themselves and each other. Only then can they effectively meet the challenges resulting from the impact of the epidemic. New information suggests that between 12 and 13 African women are currently infected for every 10 African men. HIV/AIDS is a gender issue because the risks and consequences are different for women and men:

- Women are more susceptible to HIV infection on each sexual encounter because of the biological nature of the process and the vulnerability of the reproductive tract tissues to the virus, especially in young women. Circumcision in males (not females) appears to confer some protection against Sexually Transmitted Diseases (STDs) including HIV. Men and women's risk of acquiring HIV escalates in the presence of STDs. STDs in women are more difficult to detect and thus lead to women not being easily diagnosed. The stigma of STDs in women also further reduces them accessing adequate treatment;

- Women are often less able to negotiate safer sex due to their lower status, economic dependence, fear of violence, fear of insisting on safer sex practices, etc;

- Men's sexual behaviour before or outside marriage is condoned and sometimes encouraged while that of females is repressed. This often results in social acceptance of men having sexual experimentation before marriage and extramarital relationships. Thus different rules apply for men and women which women are often unable to challenge or change;

- Young women and girls are increasingly being targeted for sex by older men seeking safe partners or where there is a belief that one can be cleansed from HIV by having sex with such women;

- Women known to have HIV/AIDS are more likely to be rejected, expelled from the family home, denied treatment, care and basic human rights.

In many ways the inequity that women and girls suffer as a result of HIV/AIDS serves as a barometer of their general status in society and the discrimination they encounter in the health field.

Commonwealth Response to HIV/AIDS

The nine most heavily infected countries in the world are Commonwealth countries. The Commonwealth Secretariat has initiated several activities and programmes with the collaboration of UN Agencies such as the World Health Organisation to address the epidemic. The outcomes of these programmes have been brought to the attention of Heads of Government and Ministers who have given them their support and called for more efforts to be initiated. Initiatives that have already been taken, or that are currently being carried out, include the following:

- **1991:** The Commonwealth Heads of Government Meeting (CHOGM) requested the Secretariat to monitor the development of multisectoral approaches to HIV/AIDS control;

- **1994:** Development of HIV/AIDS Community Based AIDS Prevention and Control programmes in Central, Southern and West Africa;

- **1995:** The Commonwealth Youth Programme (CYP) initiated an 'Ambassadors of Positive Living' programme which provided selected youth leaders from affected countries in Africa with the skills and tools to advocate for the prevention of the spread of HIV in their communities;

- **1996:** The Commonwealth Secretariat published a report on HIV/AIDS Health Policy and Legal Aspects. The report details policy and legal aspects of HIV/AIDS and contains a survey of legislation relating to HIV/AIDS in selected Commonwealth countries;

- **1996:** CYP publication, *A Guide to Preventing HIV/AIDS and STDs among Youth*, a resource book to assist young people in developing HIV/AIDS and STD health promotion projects for their communities;

- **1997:** Regional Workshop on the Development of Health Information Systems for HIV/AIDS and STD programmes in East Africa;

- The development of resource materials to assist peer educators, *Integrating Gender Awareness into Adolescent Sexual Health Programmes*;

- **1998:** Report on the status of blood transfusion services, HIV/AIDS home care and sex education in Commonwealth countries;

- **1999:** The Commonwealth Ministers of Health at their pre-World Health Assembly (WHA) meeting in Geneva in May called for the declaration of a Global AIDS Emergency;

- **1999:** The Commonwealth Secretariat's Science and Technology Division and the Association of Commonwealth Universities Expert Group held a meeting on HIV/AIDS in the Commonwealth, which will lead to the development of a knowledge network for academics in Commonwealth universities.

The Secretariat, through its Commonwealth Fund for Technical Co-operation has made available experts and consultants to assist countries develop selected aspects of their health systems. This has led to some support to the development of HIV/AIDS programmes.

Multisectoral Response to HIV/AIDS

The global response to the epidemic has shifted over several years from a health or biomedical approach to a multisectoral response to address HIV/AIDS in a more comprehensive way using the limited resources available.

The multisectoral approach requires that analysis, priority setting and planning takes place across all sectors. Particularly important is the involvement of sectors and programmes dealing with poverty alleviation, environmental degradation, urban growth and policy. In all sectors, programmes need to deal with gender, economic power imbalances, migrations, social and economic marginalisation, development of community responses and participation, and capacity building for sustainability. These issues are critical both as determinants and consequences of the spread of HIV.

Each sector needs to determine how the spread of the HIV epidemic is caused or contributed to by issues within their own purview, and how the epidemic is likely to affect their own sector's plans, objectives and goals in the future.

Responding to HIV/AIDS: The Role of Ministries Responsible for Women's Affairs and Gender Management Systems

It is now widely accepted that the HIV/AIDS emergency requires a co-ordinated response across all sectors of government. HIV/AIDS is not just a health issue but is of concern to every sector, and each sector must establish its own contribution to assist society in combating the disease and coping with its effects. The international community, led by UNAIDS, has encouraged all countries to develop Strategic Plans. A feature of these is the establishment of National Commissions (NCs) for HIV/AIDS to organise and co-ordinate this multisectoral response. However, relatively few countries have yet established NCs that are functioning effectively.

As the lead agents for mainstreaming gender, National Women's Machineries (NWMs) can play a number of key roles in supporting the national response to HIV/AIDS and in safeguarding the position of women. Furthermore, Gender Management Systems may prove to be a useful tool in achieving these objectives.

Ministers Responsible for Women's Affairs

Ministers Responsible for Women's Affairs may wish to call on National Women's Machineries to:

- advocate for the inclusion of gender analysis as an important step in the development of multisectoral response to HIV/AIDS across sectors and provide expertise in effecting this approach;

- monitor the progress of HIV/AIDS in their countries, including its specific impact on women and girls;

- advocate for improved health education and public awareness and the adoption of all measures that will limit the transmission of the virus, including safe sex, increased use of condoms and the use of safe blood products;

- liaise with and support the work of NCs for HIV/AIDS in co-ordinating the fight against the disease through the provision of budget lines and staff for developing and implementing multisectoral responses across all sectors;

- strengthen national capacities for gender analysis and planning through improving collection of sex-disaggregated data, development of gender-sensitive indicators and creating training tools and training capacities in local institutions.

Ministers may also wish to consider how to respond to the declaration by CHOGM that AIDS is a Global Emergency. They may further wish to emphasise the need for special efforts to be made to protect the health of women exposed to the risk of HIV/AIDS and to consider measures to ensure that the legal, civil and human rights of those infected are protected and that they have full access to treatment, counselling and support on an equal footing with men.

In view of the centrality of gender, Ministers Responsible for Women's Affairs may wish to call on the Gender and Youth Affairs Division and the Human Resources Development Division to collaborate closely in evolving joint strategies to combat HIV/AIDS.

Gender Management Systems

The GMS is a set of structures and processes that are designed to co-ordinate activities across all branches of government and to provide effective machineries for the explicit insertion of gender issues into the mainstream activities of all ministries and services. In the light of these characteristics, the GMS may serve in a number of ways as a valuable tool in combating HIV/AIDS:

- Where a GMS is already being piloted in a country, it could strengthen the development of a multisectoral response to HIV/AIDS by assisting in the development of a cross-sectoral, integrated response;

- The Commonwealth experience of designing and piloting a cross-sectoral, integrated approach to gender provides an important model for applying similar approaches to other problems. Thus, even where there are no plans to implement a GMS as such, these plans may serve as a blueprint for National Commissions to follow in constructing their systems to fight HIV/AIDS.

Young People Responding to HIV/AIDS in the Commonwealth

Commonwealth Secretariat

According to a recent World Health Organisation report, HIV/AIDS is now the primary cause of disease in developing countries and is having the most destructive impact not only on death rates but also on rates of premature death and disability. HIV/AIDS is unusually catastrophic because it targets young people, and the number of deaths is accelerating quickly. AIDS has been described as a 'human development crisis'.

The participation of young people is vital to reversing the devastating impact of HIV/AIDS. Young people can talk to their peers about the dangers of HIV infection and can be heard. They are the best advocates for promoting youth-friendly clinics and are the most effective leaders in communicating prevention messages with the goal of changing behaviour.

Despite the adverse news of the spread of the HIV/AIDS epidemic and the persistence of factors that sustain its spread, there are a number of successful responses that have been conducted in many parts of the Commonwealth, indicating a real decline in HIV/AIDS among young people.

Key to these successful strategies is the commitment by governments to ensure that young people are protected and provided with opportunities to develop and exercise skills that will help them to live through the epidemic and become responsible citizens. Youth empowerment strategies need to be promoted to allow youth to take responsibility in HIV/AIDS prevention. When empowered, young people have been shown to be capable of very positive changes in their circumstances. This article will highlight some of these successes and makes recommendations for replication on a larger scale.

The Global Dimensions of the Epidemic

Over the past 10 years the HIV/AIDS epidemic has spread rapidly to all parts of the world. The majority of people living with HIV – some 95 per cent of the global total – live in developing countries. This proportion is set to grow as infection rates continue to rise in countries where factors such as poverty, poor health systems and limited resources for prevention and care contribute to the spread of the virus.

In industrialised countries the spread of the epidemic has markedly reduced. This has been achieved through a number of actions ranging from national HIV-specific prevention programmes to general promotion of social and environmental changes that reduce the vulnerability and susceptibility of individuals to acquiring HIV through risk behaviours. Despite this success there is evidence suggesting that safe sexual behaviour is being eroded among gay men in some Western countries, probably due to a complacency brought about by the use of more effective antiretroviral drugs. This serves as a warning for us to avoid complacency when success is achieved and to emphasise the importance of setting in motion strategies that sustain activities that are effective against the epidemic.

The huge gap in HIV infection rates and AIDS deaths between rich and poor countries, and more particularly between Africa and the rest of the world, is likely to grow even larger in the next century. This problem can be addressed more strongly and with some certainty through increased efforts both at national and international levels. The actions that need to be carried out to achieve this end are well documented, such as ending the stifling silence that continues to surround HIV in many countries and expanding prevention initiatives such as condom promotion to reduce sexual transmission. It is essential to create conditions in which young children have the knowledge and the emotional and financial support to grow up free of HIV.

An unprecedented opportunity for wealth creation and the betterment of the human condition has been brought about by globalisation through reduced barriers to trade and enhanced capital flows for economic growth. However, the benefits of globalisation are not shared equitably and prosperity remains the preserve of the few. The persistence of poverty and human deprivation makes global peace and security fragile, limiting the growth of markets, and forcing millions to migrate in search of a better life.

The Fancourt Declaration issued at the Commonwealth Heads of Government Meeting, Durban, South Africa, November 1999, called for improved market access for exports and the removal of all barriers to the exports of the least developed countries. It also called for a reversal of the decline in official development assistance flows and action to tackle the unsustainable debt burden of developing countries. This will allow development assistance to be focused on human development, poverty reduction and on expanding world markets for goods and capital. These changes will have a beneficial impact on youth in providing a stable and enabling environment in which they can grow, having access to knowledge and emotional and financial support, free of HIV.

Gender, HIV/AIDS and Youth

Gender analysis is crucial to understanding HIV/AIDS transmission and initiating appropriate programmes of action. A number of socially constructed aspects of male-female relations underpin individual behaviour, as well as the gender-based rules, norms and laws governing the broader social and institutional context. A correct analysis thus forms the basis for the changes required to create an environment in which young people can protect themselves. Only then can they effectively meet the challenges resulting from the impact of the epidemic. Unfortunately, new information suggests that between 12 and 13 African women are currently infected for every 10 African men. This seems to emphasise the importance of recognising HIV/AIDS as a gender issue as the risks and consequences are different for women and men. These include the following:

• Young women are more susceptible to HIV infection on each sexual encounter because of the biological nature of the process and the vulnerability of the reproductive tract tissues to the virus. Circumcision in males (not females) appears to confer some protection against STDs, including HIV;

• Young women and girls are increasingly being targeted for sex by older men seeking safe partners or where there is a belief that one can be cured from HIV by having sex with such women;

• Men's sexual behaviour before or outside marriage is often condoned and sometimes encouraged while that of females is repressed. This often results in the societal acceptance of men having sexual experimentation before marriage and extramarital relationships. Different rules apply for men and women, which women are often unable to challenge or change;

• Women are often less able to negotiate for safer sex due to their lower status, economic dependence, fear of violence or fear of insisting on safer sex practices. This dominance by men is also used when initiating the sex act. Some men prefer to use force as the norm;

• The risk of acquiring HIV for both men and women escalates in the presence of STDs. STDs in women are more difficult to detect and this leads to women not being easily diagnosed. The stigma of STDs in young people, especially young women, further reduces their ability to access adequate treatment;

• Young and unmarried women known to have HIV/AIDS are more likely to be rejected, expelled from the family home and denied treatment, care and basic human rights.

Impact of HIV/AIDS on Youth

The socio-economic and political situations in a number of developing Commonwealth countries do not facilitate the control of HIV infection. The twin difficulties of unfavourable international trading conditions for primary products and non-performing economies do not allow for a positive environment in which youth are able to initiate preventive strategies in responses to the epidemic. Yet, despite these conditions, some successes have been achieved in some countries. These point to the possibilities for overcoming the epidemic in unfavourable situations and provide fresh hope for the future.

Youth in the Community

The epidemic continues to have a detrimental impact on all aspects of community life. The long time lag between HIV infection, AIDS and death – more than 10 years on average – helps to explain why most countries have yet to see the damage the epidemic can do to their social and economic fabric. The most affected age group is 15–49 years, the period when young people and adults are most productive. One of the greatest impacts is visible in sub-Saharan Africa, where the epidemic began in the late 1970s and has reached high levels of intensity. In this region, reports show that the epidemic is eclipsing health and other development gains that governments, citizens and development agencies have worked so hard to achieve. The loss of parents to AIDS leaves young people without an effective supportive social environment that is necessary for life-skills development, guidance and counselling. This loss of knowledge in communities has a detrimental effect on the choices young people make for the future.

Yuda Sanyu Kitali was 10 in 1992 when his mother died of AIDS. The disease had killed his father in 1986. Sanyu had to drop out of school as had his brother, Emmanuel Kulabigwo, now 16, and Margaret Nalubega, 15. When their parents died, they did not have any hope of affording academic fees. A year after the children were orphaned, the grass-thatched house their father had built in the Rakai district of Uganda collapsed in heavy rain. 'Since I was the eldest, I had to build another house', Sanyu says. He did his best with mud poles, reeds and banana fibre. The children grew cassava and greens on the land their parents had left them, but they still went to sleep hungry many nights.

Newsweek, 17 January 2000

Poor Economic Performance Affects Youth

AIDS affects individuals in their most productive years and leads to poor economic performance. This arises when the infected individuals develop symptomatic HIV infection resulting in the loss of productive work through absences and increased expenditure on medical and sick benefits.

The impacts are particularly severe when there are few trained individuals to carry on the work of sick workers. Their replacement with junior and inexperienced staff can lead to poor decisions or damage to equipment. Young people can be compelled to do work that they would not ordinarily do at this stage in their lives, exposing them to stress and injuries. All these factors have several consequences, including reduced savings, reinvestment or spending and finally leading to a downturn in the development of social and economic sectors. The results are poorer services for all in the community, with young people most likely to be affected as they are less well established in the community.

Initiating a Response to HIV/AIDS and Youth

Preventing new HIV infections is ultimately the best way of averting all the impacts of HIV/AIDS on youth. Success hinges on using a careful mix of tried-and-tested prevention methods. However, some initiatives such as sexual health education at school, or harm-reduction programmes for drug users, may be more costly in terms of political capital than the resources required for implementation.

A multisectoral response is also needed that is focused on youth-related activities. The multisectoral approach requires that analysis, priority setting and planning takes place across all sectors. Particularly important is the involvement of sectors and programmes dealing with poverty alleviation, environmental degradation, urban growth and policy. In all sectors programmes need to deal with gender, economic power imbalances, migration, social and economic marginalisation, development of community responses and participation and capacity building for sustainability. These issues are critical both as determinants and consequences of the spread of HIV.

Youth Ministries, in conjunction with other sectors such as Health and Education, should determine how the spread of the HIV epidemic affects issues within their own purview, and how the epidemic is likely to affect their plans, objectives and goals in the future.

At the 1995 International Conference on STD/AIDS in Kampala, Uganda, a 'delegation' of young Africans from 11 countries, ranging in age from 14 to 24, issued a declaration of their needs and priorities. The declaration put forward a series of seven principles that UNAIDS has endorsed as essential for effective AIDS action. They are still relevant for application today and the examples show that several member states have implemented them successfully.

1. Youth participation

'Involve us in programme planning, implementation and evaluation and policy develop-ment in community decision-making processes.'

As part of a report to The Pacific Youth Ministerial Meeting of 1998, a project called Youthmedia was established. This involved holding a workshop for young people in media production and distribution in Suva area, Fiji Islands. Two major radio stations and both English language daily newspapers supported the initiative by donating air time and/or column space on a weekly basis for four weeks. The young people identified topics such as pressure, unemployment, substance abuse and sexual health to be addressed through radio and television programmes.

The programme was very successful both for the young people who participated in it and their intended audience. The group is now being used by UNICEF, the Fiji Government Secretariat for the South Pacific and others to inform their pro-gramme and policies.
Source: Force for Change, UNAIDS/99.45E 1999.

Along similar lines to the Malawi Youth Council, the UN partners against AIDS in the country have established a UN youth theme group. This provides capacity building for the Malawi Youth Council and helps implement AIDS activities. It has also helped bring the voices of young people to policy makers and decision-makers.

The Uganda AIDS Commission co-ordinated the involvement of youth in the World AIDS campaign at national level by ensuring that young people participate alongside government departments, NGOs and UN agencies and others. This has resulted in the formation of a policy proposal on young people and HIV/AIDS.
Source: Force for Change, UNAIDS/99.45E 1999.

2. Youth friendly services

'Support the provision of services including centres where we can access information, support and referral.'

In Ghana, the Salvation Army has played a central role in promoting the involvement of youth in the creation of numerous projects on sex education and the provision of mobile youth STD/HIV/AIDS clinics providing treatment, health education and counselling for youth. A youth drama group has also been created which performs at youth rallies initiating discussion about abstinence and safer sex practice.

Small group discussions called 'community conversations' have brought together young people to discuss issues such as HIV/AIDS and behavioural and cultural practices that increase risk. These groups have been useful for advising policy makers on action at national level.

The West Africa Project to Combat AIDS and STDs in Adabraka, Ghana, promoted the use of condoms among sex workers and other outreach activities. A successful outcome of this is an increase in the accessibility of STD clinics to young people and the training of clinic staff in the management of STD/HIV/AIDS cases.
Source: Force for Change, UNAIDS/99.45E 1999.

3. Parental involvement

'Strengthen the capacity of parents and other significant persons in our lives to better communicate with us and provide guidance and support to us, our brothers and sisters.'

The Mathare Sports Youth Association (MYSA) was started in 1987 with the aim of addressing environmental clean ups in Nairobi, Kenya. It has also developed a strong AIDS prevention initiative over the years.

Since its inception it was unable to enlist the participation of girls in football for several years. This was because boys scoffed at the idea of girls playing football, parents felt that football was not for girls and in any case their daughters were needed at home to look after younger siblings, help with cooking, fetch water and do laundry. Moreover, many girls themselves lacked the self-confidence to try playing football.

In 1992 MYSA put together a three-year project to involve girls in its activities. Three young men who were experienced players and coaches agreed to organise the girls. Often this involved the delicate task of visiting girls' parents to convince them that their daughters were safe with MYSA. The number of girls participating has increased steadily over the years and today it has one of the largest number of girls in a youth football club in Africa.

Source: Youth to Youth – HIV prevention and young people in Kenya, Strategies for Hope Series No 13, 1997.

4. Education about HIV/AIDS and sexuality

'Promote skills based on physical development, reproductive health and sexuality for both in and out of school youth.'

At the end of 1998 in New Delhi, India, the Department of Youth and the Nehru Yuva Kendra, a national NGO, in collaboration with UNICEF India, held a 3-day planning workshop for HIV/AIDS prevention programmes for rural youth.

The Indian National Department of Education, the National AIDS Control Organisation, the National Centre for Education Research and Training, UNESCO and UNICEF conducted a workshop for the finalisation of a 16 state-level plan for the introduction of HIV/AIDS preventive education in schools.

Source: Force for Change, UNAIDS/99.45E 1999.

5. Protection of girls and young women

'Prevent the sexual abuse and exploitation of girls in vulnerable situations; emphasise the sensitisation of boys, young men and elderly men.'

A study by UNAIDS on the impact of HIV and sexual health education on sexual behaviour of young people has identified the important role of educating men about their sexuality:

Gender does not simply equate with women; it concerns men as well. It is clear from every country studied that young men are sadly neglected by families and societies when it comes to their sexuality and sexual development.

For all their sexual activity, for all the instances of sexual distress and anguish they inflict on young women, young men pursue sex and are left to pursue sex and their understanding of it in almost total silence and the absence of support. It is not surprising therefore that they get it wrong so often. There is a clear need to demarcate a specific agenda for young men in addition to that for young women which is already established.

Source: UNAIDS Best Practice Collection. Geneva, Switzerland, 1999.

6. Partnership with people with HIV and AIDS

'Build networks between young people with HIV/AIDS and other youth to promote the prevention of HIV/AIDS, protection of human rights and acceptance of people with HIV/AIDS in the society.'

7. Young people's commitments

'We commit ourselves to responsible decision-making about our own sexual behaviour and positively influence our peers.'

Since it was set up in 1996, the Botswana YMCA's Peer Approach to Counselling by Teens (PACT) has been successful in achieving its goal of empowering youth (both male and female) with knowledge and skills that will enhance their self-esteem and build positive, holistic, responsible individuals with a well-defined value system who can make informed decisions in important areas of their lives and positively influence their peers.

Tshepo, a 17-year-old girl in form III at Mater Sepi College in Francistown, has this to say about PACT:

I used to be a naughty student, I liked playing around and doing all sorts of things. My teacher told me to join PACT club, so I went along and joined in. I liked the way students were self-confident and active. After some training with PACT my attitude changed and now I am able to help other students, mostly girls, with boyfriend troubles. Since joining I have become confident and I am not afraid of anything or anyone.

Source: A Common Cause – Young people, sexuality and HIV/AIDS in three African countries. Strategies for Hope Series No 12, 1997.

Acknowledgement

This material was originally presented at the conference, 'The HIV/AIDS Crisis: A Commonwealth Response', Marlborough House, London, 7 December 2000.

Controversy, Stigma and Education: Media Coverage of HIV/AIDS in the Commonwealth

Martin Foreman

Given that the AIDS-related issues of sex and death arouse strong emotions, it is hardly surprising that coverage of the disease by the Commonwealth media has frequently been associated with controversy. Controversy itself is not harmful, but in the case of AIDS it is often accompanied by condemnation and hostility. The impact of such stigma is severe; it discourages those with HIV or at risk of contracting the virus from seeking support and advice, particularly in regard to adopting safer sex measures. Put bluntly, stigma enables AIDS to spread.

In Australia, Canada, New Zealand and the United Kingdom ('AuCaNZUK') in the 1980s, and elsewhere in the Commonwealth in the 1990s, stigma implicitly or explicitly dominated news coverage of HIV/AIDS. While stigmatisation continues in the popular press, many newspapers now focus on the social causes and consequences of the epidemic, an approach which, by demystifying the disease, implicitly combats stigma. Meanwhile, the entertainment media are in a strong position to educate the public about HIV/AIDS and similarly encourage inclusion of those affected. In some countries the entertainment media take this role seriously; in others they appear more reticent.

Mirrors and Magnifiers

The media play a central role in the lives of Commonwealth citizens. This is particularly true for those who live in urban areas and have easy access to radio and television, newspapers and magazines. But even those deprived of direct contact with the media – due to illiteracy, poverty or lack of electricity – are indirectly influenced by the programmes and articles that others watch or read. Indeed, the more restricted the media, the more closely they are identified with a society's perception of itself and the greater the influence they have on disseminating information and opinion.

That does not mean that the media are somehow separate from society, imposing alien ideas on an unsuspecting public. It is rare that newspapers, radio or television alone define public attitudes on any topic, whether HIV/AIDS or foreign policy, sport or the private lives of celebrities. Unless it is supported by government or private monopoly, any periodical or broadcast station that ignores or overrides its audience's core beliefs soon loses that audience. The media usually reflects or magnifies already existing opinions; only occasionally do they consciously try to change those opinions. In most cases, therefore, analysis of the media is by implication also an analysis of public opinion.

Stigma in the News Media

It is when the media act as a magnifying glass, exaggerating existing prejudices and ignorance, that they most obviously fuel stigma. In reporting AIDS, the popular press in particular, driven by the goal of selling as many copies as possible, has generally sought the most sensationalist headline, photograph and approach. In AuCaNZUK, sensationalism was most often seen in the early 1980s, highlighting gay[1] aspects of the disease; 'Fourth "gay plague" suspect reported' (*The Australian*, 26 May 1983) was a typical headline at the time. Awareness that most gay men are not HIV-positive, and that the epidemic is far worse elsewhere, gradually reduced the incidence of such stereotyping. Yet the influence of the media is seen over a decade later as the equation 'Gay = AIDS = Death' is still held to be true by a few individuals in these four countries.

In the mid-1980s the realisation that there was a serious AIDS epidemic in Africa moved the focus of stigma. 'Doomsday reports shock Whitehall: African AIDS "deadly threat to Britain"', reported the British *Daily Telegraph* on 20 September 1986. Not surprisingly, the response in those countries which felt themselves attacked by such headlines was hostility and denial. 'AIDS: western bias smacks of racism', stated the *Kenya Times* on 4 December 1986.

An effective response to the epidemic in East Africa was certainly delayed by several years, at least in part as backlash to the portrayal of the region in the northern media. It remains speculative as to whether a less sensationalist approach would have allowed a quicker response to AIDS. What is not speculative, however, is the long-term impact of such reporting; even today a few Africans persist in believing that the disease does not exist or is in some way a western plot.

Denial of the epidemic was not restricted to Africa. Throughout the 1980s the belief prevailed in South Asia that that region was more 'moral' and that only a few individuals would contract HIV/AIDS. With hindsight, it is easy to see that this view was short-sighted. Investigative journalism, the media's forte, failed; few journalists in India undertook the research that would have revealed the high rate of sexually transmitted infections, flourishing brothels, widespread sex between men and, in some places, high rates of drug injection that allowed the epidemic to spread.

If the possibility of an indigenous epidemic was ignored in India, the African epidemic was not. A 1986 government edict, reissued the following year, required universities to test all foreign students for HIV and expel those with the virus. This led to some Indian newspapers naming those found positive. A few others criticised the Government stance – 'an example of unwisdom' (*Chandigarh Tribune*), 'a panic reaction' (*Hindustan Times*), 'ill thought out, insensitive and blatantly discriminatory' (*Times of India*)[2] – which may have gone some way towards calming public opinion. Nonetheless, the damage was done. There were demonstrations and protests by African students, who alleged that they were being segregated both inside and outside their places of study. According to one report, the personal effects of at least one African with HIV were ordered to be burnt and many others, voluntarily or otherwise, returned home before their studies were completed.

While the media fuelled stigma against Africans and gay men, it did not create it. Prejudice tends to flourish where it already exists. Otherwise American ex-servicemen would have been blamed for Legionnaires' Disease, which was first identified in that group. But even when the media's attention moves elsewhere, the fear of AIDS is such that stigmatisation affects all those associated with the disease – and that stigma is long-lasting and can be fatal.

In Bangladesh in early 1994, two men who tested positive for HIV left their villages in fear of their lives after their names were printed in a leading newspaper. Five years later in the same country, *Bhorer Kagoj* (30 September 1999) reported that a man was confined to a bamboo cage by his fellow villagers because initial (but not subsequent) tests suggested he had HIV. The article reported the incident and pointed out that the reaction in the village was unnecessary and extreme. In South Africa, Gugu Dlamini was beaten to death by neighbours in December 1998 after she had announced on radio and television that she was living with HIV. The media might have moved on – but public awareness has not.

Working with the Media

It has taken time for the media to change its style of reporting HIV. After all, it is argued, newspapers publish the names of competition winners, of the victims of car accidents, of convicted criminals and everyone else in the news; since AIDS is newsworthy, why should those living with the virus not be treated in the same way? (Several answers are possible, starting with the fact that an individual's medical condition should be confidential.)

Partly in response to such arguments, and partly to help the media inform the general public and policy makers about the underlying causes and consequences of the disease, considerable efforts have been made to train reporters, particularly in the worst affected countries, on how to cover the disease.

Media training, organised by a range of organisations, including UN agencies and the Panos Institute, takes different forms. These include meetings, handbooks and fellowships whereby journalists receive both funding and advice to report on AIDS for a specific project or period of time. In the early 1990s, to dispel the myth that HIV is transmitted through insects or casual contact, training tended to emphasise transmission and prevention facts. In the late 1990s, training focused more on the social causes of AIDS – poverty, inequalities between men and women, and cultural factors which prevent many individuals from protecting themselves and their partners. Throughout the decade, there was implicit or explicit discussion of the conflicting goals and ethics of reporting HIV – the extent to which journalists should or should not be health educators and the impact that reporting has on the public's responses to the epidemic.

These activities have left their mark and in many Commonwealth countries there has been a marked increase in the quality of reporting on the issue. There is still sensationalism, since commercial forces are often much stronger than the impulse to act as public health educators, but this has been significantly reduced.

Yet although there is overall improvement, problems remain. In south Asia there is the impression among many professionals that the issue has been covered enough. There is also a diminishing interest in health stories and a feeling that journalists who regularly attend AIDS workshops or receive fellowships have jumped on a foreign-driven bandwagon whose interests may not coincide with those of their own country. In Africa, where the epidemic is never far from the headlines, the standard of reporting is not always high. Talented journalists have little incentive to stay in a poorly paid profession and those who remain have little formal training and limited incentive to perform well. As a result, some articles are inappropriate – such as the half-page in the *Times of Zambia* on 12 September 1999 which claimed that AIDS was created by agents of the devil and a cure had been discovered by a New Zealand preacher in 1989. While the same newspaper carried good articles on the subject on subsequent pages, it was depressing to those who had come to Lusaka to attend an international conference on AIDS in Africa that the first story in Zambia's leading newspaper was full of falsehoods, illogicalities and inconsistencies.

But such failures are not confined to one country or one continent. For several years in the early 1990s, the British *Sunday Times*, for reasons best known to its editor, maintained that AIDS was not caused by HIV and that there was no evidence for the epidemic in Africa. In other papers, reporters have complained that their expertise in HIV/AIDS is not recognised by editors who are not interested in the topic. And sometimes well-written articles are distorted by sub-editors seeking the most newsworthy, rather than the most informative, angle.[3]

Information through Entertainment

While the Commonwealth news media, particularly the press, have regularly covered AIDS, the entertainment media, predominantly radio and television, sometimes appear more reluctant to do so. This is only partly explained by the fact that producers of programmes and magazines that focus on music and drama seldom see their role as health educators. Denial or reluctance to deal with the issue also plays a part. Yet AIDS is as much a social as a medical phenomenon and there are many opportunities for scriptwriters of television or radio soap operas and dramas to bring up the subject, particularly when plotlines cover such issues as infidelity, poverty, prostitution or drug injection.

AIDS has appeared in the popular British television soap, *EastEnders* and the South African serial, *Soul City*. *EastEnders* exists primarily to entertain, while *Soul City* receives grants from a number of agencies to cover public health and other issues, but both programmes regularly include storylines that are designed to inform their audience in a non-didactic way. With AIDS, scriptwriters worked with experts to produce plots that not only provided drama but educated their audiences as to how HIV is or is not transmitted. Furthermore, by making the characters who were either infected or affected by the virus sympathetic, the scriptwriters implicitly and explicitly tackled the question of stigmatisation.

That does not mean there has been no mention of AIDS outside drama. In many countries public service announcements produced by AIDS organisations have been broadcast on all kinds of state or private networks. Individual programmes or programme hosts have included AIDS as a topic on talk shows and programmes directed at specific audiences, such as women, or rural communities. There is nevertheless scope for much more coverage of AIDS as a social issue with specific problems and a range of possible solutions.

And Now?

The extent to which AIDS will be covered by the media in the next decade is uncertain. It is likely to remain high in the priorities of the news media, as issues such as the socio-economic impact of the disease and the cost of providing access to treatment remain on the political agenda. With the entertainment media, however, the negative aspects of AIDS may keep it at a distance.

Television is a case on its own. 'Doordarshan', the Indian State broadcasting company, has been widely accused of ignoring the issue of AIDS. This apparent reluctance to include the topic in programming is at least partly a consequence of the ongoing communications revolution. In almost every Commonwealth country, the arrival of multiple television channels, by satellite or cable, has led to either a severe fall in public service broadcasting or a fall in the proportion of the overall audience watching such programmes. As station goals focus more on audience numbers than on content, AIDS educators find it difficult to provide accurate, informative input into television. In contrast, despite the multiplication of radio stations, it appears easier for AIDS to be covered, as talk show hosts in the Caribbean, news reporters in Africa and public service broadcasters in Asia all indicate a wish to keep the issue prominent in their programmes.

How much the internet will influence coverage of HIV is still unclear. As a proportion of the population, up to 100 times more people in the United Kingdom than in India can go on-line, but that does not mean that Britons consider the internet their primary source of information. What is certain is that the news media themselves are making increasing use of the net. Nigeria has seen the development of several on-line networks, such as Nigeria-AIDS, which provide journalists with information about the latest statistics, discoveries and pronouncements both nationwide and worldwide. 'AF-AIDS' and 'SEA-AIDS' serve English-speaking Africa, and south and south-east Asia, respectively, bringing together not only the media, but all those working in AIDS prevention and care in those regions, while 'Health-L' [Zambia] and 'Shohojogi-AIDS' perform a similar service in Zambia and Bangladesh. Access to information does not in itself solve the problem of quality, but the very existence of such networks does provide some form of quality control, as new ideas are debated and those which are found wanting are rejected.

Notes

1. In this article, 'gay' refers to men who acknowledge their sexual attraction to other men – a small minority in the Commonwealth in comparison with the numbers of men who, regularly or occasionally, voluntarily or under compulsion, have sex with other men.

2. Other than the year 1987, the dates of these extracts are not available to the writer.

3. Although not related to this discussion, a prime example of subversion by subediting appeared in the British *Daily Mail* in the early 1990s. An informative article on a possible genetic cause of male homosexuality was headlined 'Abortion hope after gene finding', despite the fact that abortion was not mentioned in the article.

Regional Impacts and Responses

Sexually Transmitted Diseases: An Asian Perspective

Lalit K Bhutani and Neena Khanna

Sexually Transmitted Diseases (STDs) are some of the commonest causes of illness in Asia and several other parts of the world. The introduction of penicillin and other antibiotics in medicine gave rise to a fond hope that control of STDs was around the corner. The continuing rise in the number of patients with STDs in the world, and particularly in Asia and Africa, betrayed the fact that antibiotics alone would not be effective against a group of infections in which a basic human (and animal) instinct, namely sex, was the predominant mode of transmission. Introduction of HIV infection and the emergence of a potentially fatal disease, AIDS, jolted the medical profession and the world at large out of a state of complacency. Brundtland[1] observed:

HIV affects more people than it infects. It makes families poor as they try to meet the cost of health care – poorer as they cope with the loss of income following the death of a bread-winner. HIV leaves behind orphans with uncertain futures.

Asia, home to almost half the world's population, has proved a fertile soil for HIV infection.

Sexual Culture

Despite religious, socio-cultural, economic and ethnic diversity in various countries of Asia, certain perceptions about sex and sexuality are common: sex is dirty and any discussion of sexuality is taboo. The paradox and dichotomy are nowhere more in evidence than in India where the symbol of (pro)creation, the Shiva-lingum (the phallus of Lord Shiva, the traditional Hindu Lord of Creation), is worshipped, and where *Kamasutra*, the gospel of the art of love-making, was written, but where any discussion of sex and sexuality is looked down upon.

Sex education, at home or at school, is limited or non-existent. What little information, or misinformation, is gained is picked up from equally ill-informed or mis-informed peers, or from cheap and vulgar pornographic literature published and sold in a clandestine manner. The situation is aggravated by self-professed 'sex doctors' whose greed for money makes them further mislead the group that needs education and information most – the gullible youth. Traditionally, loss of semen is equated with loss of vitality; masturbation and nocturnal emissions are said to be weakening – physically, sexually and mentally![2,3] On the other hand, it is also believed in some cultures that semen benefits a woman's vigour and complexion.[3]

Gender bias, namely male domination, present the world over, is in great evidence in Asia. Sex with several partners is a way of proving sexual masculinity and manhood. The female, the passive recipient of sex and a docile donor of sexual pleasures, is supposed to hold out for rewards, financial or marital.

Sexual Behaviour

Reliable data about sexual practices are not available. The information in this article has been gathered from hospital and field practices and from a few small studies carried out in a limited manner. Virginity is expected in both sexes; its loss is often overlooked in men but is unpardonable in women. Premarital and extra-marital sex is condemned and yet perhaps more widely practised than generally assumed; the same holds for homosexuality. This is often the case with men for whom sex with prostitutes is an accepted part of premarital and extramarital sexual activity in certain societies. Religion also seems to play a role in certain countries. Homosexuality is regarded as a felony in Islam and is condemned in other religions. Polygamy is sanctioned in Islam, but premarital and extramarital sex are (in Malaysia) punishable by imprisonment or fine in the case of Muslims.[4] Homo-sexuality is a criminal offence in Singapore and can attract imprisonment from two years to life. The topic of lesbianism is seldom even mentioned. Loss of chastity – voluntary or forced – may drive women to prostitution.[5] As traditional values give way, the perception about sex is being replaced by permissiveness, particularly among the youth.

Analysis of data from STD clinics in India[2] and a study in Singapore[3] show that the average age of first sexual intercourse is under 30 years of age. In the Singapore study 96 per cent of women were found to be monogamous while 46 per cent of sexually active men had more than one sexual partner. In another study from India[5] 46 per cent of women had premarital sex; this study may not reflect the true picture since it included women from tribal areas where trial marriages and sexual freedom enjoy social sanction. In Malaysia[4] half of the youth (17–24 years old) sur-veyed had experienced premarital sex. In a survey in Hong Kong[6] 48.5 per cent of males and 26.3 per cent of females admitted to premarital sex.

The differences between the sexual behaviour of males and females are striking. In the Hong Kong study, males had a 5.5 times higher high-risk activity compared to females. In Malaysia, amongst those who had 'dated', 26 per cent of boys but only 5 per cent of girls had had sexual intercourse. In Singapore 16 per cent of men had extramarital sex; the figure for women, on the other hand, was reported to be 0.1–0.2 per cent. Common situations where men are more likely to engage in extramarital relationships are driving trucks on long routes, extended travels on business and living in cities away from their families. The irony is that men who indulge more frequently in high-risk behaviour carry infection back to their wives who, while monogamous, suffer disproportionately from HIV infection and com-plications of STDs.

Commercial Sex

Prostitution is alleged to be the oldest profession in the world and continues to exist in all parts of the world including Asia – with or without legal sanction. In Malaysia voluntary prostitution by adult non-Muslims is not a crime. In India and Malaysia it is illegal to solicit prostitution though pimps are a common sight in all the red-light districts of the metropolitan cities. Commercial sex workers are either locals or immigrants from neighbouring countries. Poverty is the main, but not the sole, reason for taking to prostitution. There may be other factors too: a woman may be forced into prostitution by society after she has been raped; *devdasis* (hand-maidens) in India and *devkis* in Nepal are given away as an offering to goddesses. Women may also take up prostitution merely to supplement other income or to buy protection.

Burden of STDs

In the south-east Asia region, STDs are one of the two top-ranking communicable diseases causing loss of life measured as disability-adjusted-life-years (DALYs) lost.[7] The burden is much higher amongst females because of the complications; sequelae of STDs are most pronounced in the poorest females and in the least developed parts of Asia. The complications are the result of delay in seeking treatment and ascent of infection along the reproductive tract resulting in pelvic inflammatory disease (PID) which, in turn, may result in infertility, ectopic pregnancies, foetal wastage, still births and even maternal mortality.

Both sexes are, of course, affected in their reproductive and economically most productive period. Further, the presence of STDs, and particularly the ulcerative forms, predispose both sexes to acquisition of HIV infection 4–10 times more frequently.

Epidemiology of STDs

The epidemiology of STDs in Asia is ill-understood for a variety of socio-cultural and economic reasons. Case-notification is poor and the few epidemiological studies are inadequate for meaningful conclusions. The methods employed for studying the epidemiology are different from country to country, making comparisons difficult. STDs are not notifiable in Hong Kong. In Singapore[3] only four STDs, syphilis, gonorrhoea, non-specific urethritis and chancroid, are notifiable, since 1976, under the Infectious Diseases Act. In Malaysia[4] the Prevention and Control of Infectious Diseases Act requires only three STDs, gonorrhoea, syphilis and chancroid, to be notified The bane of studies of the incidence and prevalence of STDs is under-reporting. This is partly inherent in the nature of the diseases and partly caused by the asymptomatic nature of some of the diseases, particularly in females. Again, only a small fraction of patients attend designated STD clinics because of the stigma, lack of confidentiality and judgmental attitude of the staff at the clinics. Most patients continue to be treated by private practitioners, practitioners of alternative systems of medicine, pharmacies and pharmacists, and quacks. These patients often go unreported. In Malaysia, for instance, while most notifications come from government clinics, private practitioners see 75 per cent of patients. The problem is therefore almost always projected lower than its actual existence. This infuses less than optimum enthusiasm amongst the planners and the policy-makers.

The World Health Organisation estimated that in 1995[7] there were 333 million cases, globally, of gonorrhoea, syphilis, chlamydia and trichomoniasis. South and south-east Asia accounted for the largest number of new infections (150.8 million, or 45.6 per cent). Of these, 120 million were in the 15–49 age group. A breakdown by disease also indicated that this region contributed about half the patients. Syphilis, for instance, contributed 5.8 million patients out of a total of 12 million; 29 million patients had gonorrhoea out of a total of 62 million; 40 million had chlamydial infection out of a total of 89 million; and 75 million had trichomaniasis out of a total of 170 million. The sex distribution was skewed in favour of females – 55 per cent of cases of syphilis, 58 per cent of gonorrhoea, 60 per cent of chlamydia and 92 per cent of trichomoniasis occurred in females.

The epidemiology of STDs in the continent of Asia is very uneven and marked regional differences exist. In India the annual incidence of all STDs was estimated to affect around 5 per cent of the population – or 40 million new infections annually. In Sri Lanka the estimated number of patients is 200,000–250,000. The data from antenatal clinics seem to suggest an increasing incidence of STDs; VDRL seropositivity increased from 0.6 per cent in 1980 to 1.8 per cent in 1994 though, curiously, the incidence of gonorrhoea went down – from 20 per 100,000 in 1984 to 2 per 100,000 in 1994. The incidence of chlamydia and genital herpes seemed to be increasing.

In Hong Kong, the epidemiological pattern of STDs is inferred from the data col-lected by the Social Hygiene Service of the Department of Health, even though it is believed that only a third or a quarter of STD patients attend the clinic. This is an inadequate substitute for epidemiological studies but is the best information available on the subject.

The number of female patients reporting, in most STD clinics is small because of stigmatisation and the judgmental attitude of the staff, physicians not excluded. Many women also suffer from asymptomatic infections and thus do not report on their own; contact tracing is almost non-existent in most parts of Asia.

Singapore[3] presents a refreshing contrast from most of the other Asian countries. Accurate data on the four notifiable diseases have been available since 1977 and there is a steady decline in these STDs. Figure 1 indicates the trend.

Table 1. Profile of STDs in Social Hygiene Clinics, Hong Kong, 1986–95

	1986	1987	1988	1989	1990	1991	1992	1993	1994	1995
Syphilis	525	490	398	382	370	310	421	459	384	382
Gonorrhoea	5008	6035	4919	3075	2487	2996	2825	2754	2521	2300
NSGI/NGU	3070	3309	4819	4075	3434	4330	5293	5675	6190	8281
Chancroid	370	184	137	56	32	44	47	21	8	7
LGV	14	17	32	19	8	12	10	7	5	2
Genital herpes	370	731	919	834	762	584	719	779	766	796
Genital warts	1854	2195	2330	2007	1727	1810	1666	1898	2418	2955
Ped pubis	283	367	474	397	304	314	309	298	357	408
Others	314	793	759	1646	1333	2046	1867	1895	2199	2984
Total	11808	14184	14787	12491	10457	12446	13257	13786	14838	18115

Source: Sexually Transmitted Diseases in Asia and Pacific[6]

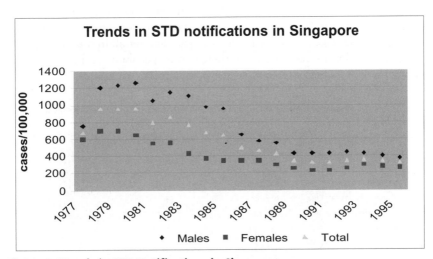

Figure 1. Trends in STD Notifications in Singapore
Source: Sexually Transmitted Diseases in Asia and Pacific[3]

HIV/AIDS and STDs

HIV infection can be transmitted through penetrative, homo- or heterosexual, relationships. It can also be acquired through penetrative injury with blood-contaminated needles, infusion of infected blood or blood products, or from the transplacental route from an infected mother to the foetus. Since a sexual route has been considered as the most frequent method of transmission, the disease it causes, namely AIDS, has been classified as an STD.

There are several features common to or inter-related between HIV/AIDS and conventional STDs. The predominant mode of transmission for both is sexual. Both groups of diseases affect the young, sexually active and economically most productive sections of the population. The presence of any STD predisposes to the acquisition and transmission of HIV infection. And the presence of concomitant HIV infection not only modifies the natural course of other STDs such as genital herpes, chancroid and syphilis, but also makes treatment that much more difficult. Effective management of STDs, on the other hand, has been shown to reduce the transmission, and thus incidence, of HIV infection.

Strategies for Prevention and Control of STDS

Control of STDs has become emergent since the spread of potentially fatal HIV infection is fuelled by people with Sexually Transmitted Infections (STIs) and people who have unprotected sex with multiple partners.[1] The traditional approach of treating a patient presenting in the clinic will no longer be effective to control either STDs or HIV infection. In the first instance, as the following figure shows, it is ultimately a very small percentage of infected individuals who are able to get to the stage of treatment, cure and patient referral. In the second, there is so much time lost in the process that there is every possibility of the patient contracting the HIV infection, so a most important opportunity is lost.

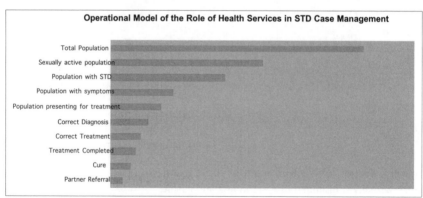

Figure 2. Operational Model of the Role of Health Services in STD Case Management
Source: Control of Sexually Transmitted Disease

Control programmes for STDs must be tailored to the individual needs of a country, based on epidemiological, socio-cultural and economic factors. The primary objectives of the control programme should be to:

- interrupt the transmission of sexually acquired infections;
- prevent the development of diseases, complications and sequelae;
- prevent the acquisition of HIV infection.

All efforts should be directed towards achieving these three objectives.

Primarily through the process of information, education and communication (IEC) people at different levels (for example, in the community, selected high-risk behaviour groups and patients presenting in the clinic) should be targeted in an attempt to interrupt STIs. Use of culturally acceptable methods of 'safe sex' must be promoted: a mutually faithful monogamous relationship, non-penetrative sex or the consistent use of condoms are some examples of safe sex. Abstinence, a most effective means of control of STDs, is much less likely to be practised than the use of condoms.

The STD control programme should be able to provide inexpensive but quality condoms at convenient sites. Use of condoms by a person with high-risk behaviour is likely to have a most significant effect. Brundtland[1] points out: 'ensuring regular use of condom by a person who has 1000 partners a year is likely to be much more efficient at reducing HIV infection than ensuring condom use by 1000 people who have one new partner a year'.

Prevention of complications and sequelae can be achieved by early and effective treatment. With the adoption of an algorithm-based syndromic approach most of the case-management problems, such as delay in making an accurate diagnosis and instituting an appropriate therapy, would be resolved. It is essential, however, that the treatment be made available in a non-stigmatising setting and that confidentiality and privacy are assured. The management must also take into account the treatment of the sexual partner and the affordability of the treatment. This could also be a good opportunity for counselling but not for judgmental sermons.

Effective prevention and control of STDs will go a long way in controlling the transmission of HIV/AIDS.

Conclusions

The scenario for STDs in Asia at present does not evoke great optimism. It is necessary for the health professionals to project accurate data in correct perspective so that policy makers and planners are made aware of the gravity of the situation. Thailand and Sonagachi (Calcutta, India) are examples of success stories where intervention by peer educators and safe sex practices have brought down the incidence of STDs. It is time for action before Asia goes the way of Africa as far as STD/HIV/AIDS are concerned.

Addendum

Since the preparation of this paper, data have been made available on VDRL and HIV sero-positivity on donors[9] (voluntary and replacement) reporting to the Blood Bank of the All India Institute of Medical Sciences, New Delhi, India (the information for 1997–2000 has kindly been provided by Dr. Ambika Nanu as an unpublished personal communication). The results are as follows.

Table 2. Donor screening: percentage seropositivity

Year	HIV (elisa)	VDRL	Total donors screened
1989	0.04	0.36	12,411
1990	0.06	0.23	12,897
1991	0.14	0.29	15,580
1992	0.22	0.31	16,558
1993	0.27	0.38	18,576
1994	0.41	0.49	18,122
1995	0.55	0.52	16,817
1996	0.39	0.35	21,132
1997	0.22	0.13	23,155
1998	0.34	0.29	23,149
1999	0.30	0.23	21,071
2000	0.28	0.59	23,222

Seropositivity for HIV has significantly gone up in later years, from 0.04 per cent and 0.06 per cent in 1989 and 1990 respectively. No consistent pattern is, however, discernible between 1992 to 2000 to permit any definite conclusions to be drawn. VDRL positivity also did not show any consistent variations. VDRL and seropositivity for HIV were significantly less frequent in voluntary donors compared to replacement donors.

References

1. Brundtland, G H (2000). 'Outstanding Issues in the International Response to HIV/AIDS: the WHO Perspective', *Journal of Health Management* 2: 151–8.

2. Khanna, N, Nadkarni, V and Bhutani, L K (1998). In Brown T, Chan R, Mugrditchian D et al. (eds). *Sexually Transmitted Diseases in Asia and the Pacific*. Melbourne: Venereology Publishing, pp. 114–37.

3. Chan, R K W, Goh, C L, Wong, M L and Chew S K (1998). In Brown, T, Chan R, Mugrditchian, D et al. (eds). *Sexually Transmitted Diseases in Asia and the Pacific*. Melbourne: Venereology Publishing, pp. 280–97.

4. Ngeow, Y F, Rus, S C and Deva, M (1998). In Brown, T, Chan, R, Mugrditchian, D et al. (eds). *Sexually Transmitted Diseases in Asia and the Pacific*. Melbourne: Venereology Publishing, pp. 162–77.

5. Bang, R A (1989). 'High prevalence of gynaecological diseases in rural Indian women', *Lancet*, 14 January (8629): 85–88.

6. Saw, T A, Lo, K K, Lee, S S and Chong, L Y (1998). In Brown, T, Chan, R, Mugrditchian D et al. (eds). *Sexually Transmitted Diseases in Asia and the Pacific*. Melbourne: Venereology Publishing pp. 102–12.

7. Gerbase, A C, Rowley, J T and Mertens, T E (1998). 'Global Epidemiology of Sexually Transmitted Diseases', *Lancet* 351 Suppl III: 2–4.

8. Dallabetta, G, Field, M L, Laga, M and Islam, M Q. 'STDs: Global Burden and Challenges for Control'. In *Control of Sexually Transmitted Diseases*. AIDSCAP/Family Health International.

9. Nanu, A, Sharma, S P, Chatterjee, K and Jyoti, P (1997). *Markers for Transfusion-transmissible Infections in North Indian Voluntary and Replacement Blood Donors: Prevalence and Trends 1989–1996*. Vox Sang 73: 70–73.

The Canadian Response to the HIV/AIDS Epidemic

Mary Lyn Mulvihill and Michael Jacino

In Canada, HIV/AIDS remains a significant national health issue. Every day, more Canadians become infected with HIV. The HIV/AIDS epidemic has had a profound impact not only on the lives of those who have contracted HIV, but also on the lives of their partners, families, friends, colleagues and caregivers. The financial burden resulting from increased infections is matched only by the enormous human cost. The resulting challenges which lie ahead are too great and too complex for a single government or a single agency. The ability to build on partnerships already in place and to build new ones is essential if Canada is to make further progress. In May 1998, the Canadian Minister of Health launched the 'Canadian Strategy on HIV/AIDS' a new approach to address the HIV/AIDS epidemic in Canada, and has committed ongoing annual funding of $42.2 million to the initiative.

Canada's Health Care System

Canada has a predominantly publicly financed, privately delivered, health care system that is best described as an interlocking set of ten provincial and three territorial health insurance plans. Known to Canadians as 'Medicare', the system provides access to universal, comprehensive coverage for medically necessary hospital, in-patient and out-patient physician services.

The Federal Government's role in health care involves the setting and administering of national principles or standards for the health care system, assisting in the financing of provincial health care services through fiscal transfers, and fulfilling meeting standards for which it is constitutionally responsible. Other Federal Government health-related functions include health protection, disease prevention and health promotion.

HIV/AIDS in Canada – the Current Situation

To date, an estimated 55,000 to 60,000 Canadians have become infected with HIV. Of these, nearly 20,000 developed AIDS by the end of 1997, and at least 12,000 have died. The reduced numbers of HIV diagnoses in Canada over the past few years offer some encouragement, but there still exists a need for vigilance. New infections continue to occur and there are between 12,000 and 18,000 Canadians who are infected with HIV but unaware of their status.

In the decade following the first case reports in 1982, most HIV infections occurred among men who had had sex with men and people who had received infected blood and blood products. Since then, local, provincial, territorial and Federal programmes and agencies have succeeded in reducing the rate of infection in the gay and bisexual male population and stringent blood-screening standards now ensure that virtually all Canadians are safe from infection through blood supply.

Current figures indicate that HIV-positive test reports are increasing among adult women, youth, aboriginal populations and injection drug users (IDU). Men who have sex with men still account for the majority of people living with HIV/AIDS in Canada.

HIV Infection in Canada (%)

MSM	Men who have sex with men	55
IDU	Injection drug users	} 22
MSM-IDU	Male injection drug users who have sex with men	
HETERO	Heterosexuals	19
BLOOD	People infected through blood or blood products	2

Source: Bureau of HIV/AIDS and STD, LCDC, 13 November 1999

How the Canadian Health Care System Works

Canada does not have a system of 'socialised medicine' with doctors employed by the government. Most doctors are private practitioners who work in independent or group practices and enjoy a high degree of autonomy. Some doctors work in community health centres, hospital-based group practices or in affiliation with hospital out-patient departments. Private practitioners are generally paid on a fee-for-service basis and submit their service claims directly to the provincial health insurance plan for payment.

When Canadians need medical care, in most instances they go to the physician or clinic of their choice and present their health insurance card (issued to all eligible residents of a province). Canadians do not pay directly for insured hospital and physicians' services, nor are they required to fill out forms for insured services. There are no deductibles, co-payments or dollar limits on coverage for insured services.

Over 95 per cent of Canadian hospitals are operated as private non-profit entities run by community boards of trustees, voluntary organisations or municipalities. Hospitals have control of the day-to-day allocation of resources, provided they stay within the operating budgets established by the regional or provincial health authorities. Hospitals are primarily accountable to the communities they serve, not to the provincial bureaucracy.

In addition to insured hospital and physician services, provinces and territories also provide public coverage for other health services that remain outside the national health insurance framework for certain groups of the population (for example, seniors, children and welfare recipients). These supplementary health benefits often include prescription drugs, dental care, vision care, assistive equipment and appliances (prostheses, wheelchairs, etc.) to independent living and services of allied health professionals such as podiatrists and chiropractors.

Although the provinces and territories do provide some additional benefits, supplementary health services are largely privately financed and Canadians must pay privately for these non-insured health benefits. The individual's out-of-pocket expenses may be dependent on income or ability to pay. Individuals and families may acquire private insurance, or benefit from an employment-based group insurance plan, to offset some portion of the expenses of supplementary health services. Under most provincial laws, private insurers are restricted from offering coverage which duplicates that of the government programmes, but they can compete in the supplementary benefits market.

The Canadian Strategy on HIV/AIDS

The Canadian Strategy on HIV/AIDS is the direct result of extensive and unprecedented consultations which took place in the autumn of 1997 in communities across Canada to address HIV/AIDS. The Canadian Strategy was developed in collaboration with the provinces and territories, the research community, community-based organisations, at-risk groups, aboriginal communities, health care professionals, persons living with HIV/AIDS, and the private sector.

The Strategy builds on more than 15 years of HIV/AIDS research, surveillance and community development. As experience and knowledge accumulate, the Canadian Strategy remains flexible enough to forge new associations and is firm enough to establish precise, proactive solutions in the fight against HIV/AIDS.

Since Canada's first case of AIDS in 1982, improved treatment has resulted in a significant decrease in newly diagnosed AIDS cases. But the epidemic is far from over. The Strategy will aid and support the continued development of effective therapies and treatments for more than 40,000 Canadians living with HIV/AIDS.

Grounded in the principles of partnership, co-ordination, accountability and flexibility, the Canadian Strategy brings those living with HIV/AIDS closer to the treatment, support and information they need. Just as the AIDS epidemic crosses all social, economic and cultural boundaries, the Canadian Strategy covers the full complement of human experience. Strategy components address not only prevention and research but also human rights, housing, education and other vital life influencers. If education is the first line in public awareness, the front line of defence against HIV is prevention – the key factor behind all Strategy initiatives.

To maintain an effective balance of research and responsiveness, the Strategy is structured to face the current needs of high-risk populations, even while the social profile of those affected by HIV/AIDS change.

Key Canadian Partners:

Canadian Aboriginal AIDS Network

Canadian AIDS Society

Canadian Association for HIV Research

Canadian Foundation for AIDS Research

Canadian HIV/AIDS Legal Network

Canadian HIV Trials Network

Canadian HIV/AIDS Clearinghouse

Canadian International Development Agency

Canadian Treatment Advocates Council

Community AIDS Treatment Information Exchange

Correctional Service Canada

Health Canada

Interagency Coalition on AIDS and Development

International Council of AIDS Service Organisations.

Research

The Strategy funds a broad range of research activities that increase our understanding of the social, economic, biomedical, clinical and public health policy aspects of HIV/AIDS. This understanding will help improve not just HIV/AIDS treatment, but also programmes for youth at risk, family caregivers, social support networks and other groups affected by HIV/AIDS. Collaborative research continues to be the cohesive force behind research strategies. Partnerships among academic institutions, scientists, community-based organisations and government agencies keep research focused on the areas of most urgent concern.

Surveillance and Epidemiological Monitoring

Early and accurate reporting has proved to be critical to preventing and containing outbreaks of HIV and in reducing the spread of HIV/AIDS. Continual improvements to the HIV/AIDS Case Reporting Surveillance System contribute to these efforts. Achieving more rapid, sensitive and accurate data-collection systems means crossing the many dimensions of this shifting epidemic. Working in tandem with prevention efforts, the Strategy's surveillance component tracks the shifting trends of HIV infections across Canada. This work also includes a risk assessment with respect to the spread of HIV infections, determining the profile of high-risk populations, estimating the current burden of disease in Canada, tracking mortality rates and assessing the people who may be unaware of their HIV status.

Community Development and Support to NGOs

Community-based organisations are the Canadian Strategy's best example of flexibility in action. These groups are on the front line of the epidemic, moving swiftly to develop breakthrough projects that target prevention efforts and improve conditions for people living with HIV/AIDS. Maintaining an open dialogue among all people affected by HIV/AIDS is a key factor in their success. Following this tradition, the Canadian Strategy sponsors an annual National NGO Meeting held with representatives of the Policy, Co-ordination and Programmes Division of the Strategy. National HIV/AIDS organisations and other mega-projects that receive operational funding bring their creativity, knowledge and experience to the table. Integrated decision-making, collaboration and strategic planning are just some of the issues discussed. These discussions will ensure that Strategy funding is put to the most effective use.

International Collaboration

The Canadian Strategy on HIV/AIDS also recognises the importance of incorporating the international context of the pandemic into the domestic response since geographical borders do not contain the spread of HIV/AIDS. Reports that 5.6 million people around the world were newly infected with HIV in 1999 alone is evidence of this tragedy. Committed to global citizenship, the Canadian Strategy therefore engages in a multitude of international activities, premised upon the fact that acting globally can also alert Canadian agencies and departments about new and innovative approaches to fight the epidemic locally. Sharing and learning is thus the cornerstone to the international collaboration component of the Canadian Strategy on HIV/AIDS. Furthermore, the activities of the Canadian International Development Agency (CIDA) complement the international component of the Canadian Strategy. In the 1998/99 fiscal year, for example, CIDA programme funding for HIV/AIDS totalled $20 million in support of various projects, including the UNICEF Romania Project on AIDS-affected Children; a Canadian programme to combat HIV/AIDS in Francophone Africa; the Southern African AIDS Training Project; and an STD/HIV Control Project developed in Kenya with the University of Manitoba and the University of Nairobi.

Programme Components of the Canadian Strategy

Out of the consultations described above, policy directions and funding priorities were established for the Canadian Strategy. These priorities are reviewed regularly to ensure that the Strategy focuses on the areas of greatest need. The following policy directions guide the implementation of the Canadian Strategy on HIV/AIDS:

- Enhanced sustainability and integration – new approaches and mechanisms will consolidate and co-ordinate sustained national action;

- Increased focus on the most at risk – innovative strategies will target high-risk behaviour in hard-to-reach populations that are often socially and economically marginalised;

- Increased public accountability – evidence-based decision-making and ongoing reviewing and monitoring of performance against stated objectives will ensure that the Strategy continues to be relevant and responsive to the changing realities of HIV/AIDS.

Goals of the Canadian Strategy

The Canadian Strategy on HIV/AIDS has a set of clear goals:

- To prevent the spread of HIV infection;

- To find a cure;

- To find effective vaccines, drugs and therapies;

- To ensure effective care, treatment and support for persons living with HIV/AIDS, and for families, friends and caregivers;

- To minimise the impact of HIV/AIDS on individuals and communities;

- To counter the social and economic factors that increase individual and collective risk of HIV infection.

Strategy Funding

Through the consultations with national non-governmental organisations, funding priorities were also established for the Canadian Strategy. As with the policy directions and goals of the Strategy, the allocation of Strategy funds is reviewed regularly to ensure that it focuses on the areas of greatest need.

The Government of Canada contributes substantially through additional annual funding from other Federal departments and agencies such as CIDA ($17M) and the Medical Research Council of Canada (MRC) ($2M). Provincial and territorial Governments provide major support through contributions to the delivery of HIV/AIDS-related health care services, research and prevention activities. Increasingly, government departments integrate HIV/AIDS into their work.

Strategy Funding for the Current Fiscal Year ($ million)

Prevention	3.9
Community development and support to national NGOs	10.0
Care, treatment and support	4.75
Research	13.15
Surveillance	4.3
International collaboration	0.3
Legal, ethical and human rights	0.7
Aboriginal health and community development	2.6
Correctional service of Canada	0.6
Consultation, evaluation, monitoring and reporting	1.9
Total	**42.2**

Directions for the Future

The essential aim of the Canadian Strategy on HIV/AIDS is to transcend the obstacles that have enabled the disease to infect thousands of Canadians. The Strategy's pan-Canadian approach to HIV/AIDS is bringing governments closer to the disease and thus mobilising greater prevention efforts. The Strategy is not only crossing the boundaries of care-giving and research but also eliminating them. It is moving nearer to the front-lines so that local outreach can meet global collaboration. The Strategy's collective goals for 2000–2001 are based on the following facts:

- HIV/AIDS has not been eradicated in Canada and remains a critical global concern;

- New treatments may help people living with HIV/AIDS live longer but survival is not guaranteed;

- HIV infections are increasing for marginalised Canadians, while thousands of Canadians still remain unaware of their HIV status;

- HIV/AIDS reaches beyond health issues to encompass urgent social, human rights and economic challenges;

- Continued collaboration with key stakeholders in HIV/AIDS-related fields will help share advances and experiences across disciplines.

By ensuring effective care and treatment for people living with HIV/AIDS, addressing social, economic, legal and ethical issues, investing more resources in research and treatment, and developing joint strategic policies and practices among Strategy partners, we create a common vision of shared hope. In the coming year, Strategy advances will best be demonstrated through the following broad directives:

- To further mobilise national efforts to reach Canadian young people by helping overcome the barriers that place those under 25 at increased risk of HIV infection;

- To enhance Canada's role in the worldwide effort to stop the spread of HIV/AIDS and implement global lessons learned on the domestic front;

- To eradicate HIV/AIDS by augmenting Canada's national and international efforts in the development of a safe and effective vaccine against HIV;

- To expand community-based and Governmental efforts through a focus on mutual priorities, planning and activities as well as to build stronger partnerships and strategic allegiances;

- To raise cultural and social awareness in order to revitalise the fight against HIV/AIDS and end complacency;

- To advocate social, political and cultural change in concert with Canada's emerging at-risk populations such as First Nations, Inuit and Métis and other visible minorities;

- To heighten Canadian awareness of the increasing threat of HIV infection among heterosexual populations;

- To refine surveillance and research priorities in order to address disturbing trends in treatment failure rates;

- To provide greater access to current HIV/AIDS information, resources and services.

A passionate commitment to open dialogue is the essence of collaboration under the Canadian Strategy on HIV/AIDS. This exciting exchange will do more than reduce the risk of infection or improve care for people living with HIV/AIDS. It will engage society in the attempt to end the discrimination and systemic barriers that place individuals at risk and inhibit compassionate care. As Canadians enter the new millennium, the Strategy will ensure progressive gains in HIV/AIDS research, treatment and care, as well as provide a healthier existence for all citizens.

And as the Strategy evolves, Canadians everywhere will devote their collaborative efforts for a community that has nothing in common with such suffering – a world without AIDS.

Information, Education and Communication on HIV/AIDS for Female Adolescents in the African Region

Regina Cammy Shakakata

HIV/AIDS in Africa

The HIV/AIDS burden in Africa, especially in sub-Saharan Africa, remains the most acute of all health problems among all regions of the world. Two-thirds of the world's HIV-positive people are resident in sub-Saharan Africa. AIDS is the leading cause of death with more than two million Africans having died in 1998. This situation has produced negative effects on development in the sub-region as observed by Nelson Mandela in 1997 when he addressed the Economic Forum in Davos, saying that AIDS kills those on whom society relies to grow crops, work in the mines and factories, run schools and govern countries.

Peter Piot, in *Africa Lifts its Silence on AIDS* (Development Outreach, Fall 1999), gave some stunning facts about HIV/AIDS in Africa. In Zimbabwe, 50 per cent of hospital patients have HIV/AIDS symptoms. By 2005, AIDS treatment costs will have risen to a third of all government spending on health in Ethiopia, more than half in Kenya and two-thirds in Zimbabwe (about 60 per cent of the total health budget).

He further states that a World Bank study on AIDS in Tanzania estimated that AIDS will kill almost 15,000 teachers by 2010 and 27,000 by 2020. The cost of training replacement teachers has been estimated at approximately US$37.8 million. In Côte d'Ivoire, it is reported that a teacher dies from AIDS every school day. This situation is a corrosion of the nerve of development in African – education.

The picture in the private sector is equally depressing. Piot qualifies the human resource depression when he says that AIDS-related costs, including absenteeism from work, insurance and costs of recruiting and retraining replacement workers, would absorb as much as one-fifth of all profits. In Zambia, for example, Barclays Bank has been losing 36 employees every year out of 1,600, ten times the death rate at most US companies. In spite of the efforts to alleviate poverty in many African countries, not much is being achieved in this area because, at household level, households with a family member who has AIDS suffer a dramatic decrease in income, consumption and savings. In Côte d'Ivoire, family spending on school education has halved and food consumption is said to have dropped by two-fifths, while individual expenditure on health care has more than quadrupled.

It is further reported that in Uganda 11 per cent of orphans had parents who died from AIDS and that in Zambia the number is 9 per cent. In Botswana, it is estimated that a child born today has a life expectancy of 41 years when normally it would have had 71. It is frightening to think about the kind of societies that will develop in Africa when more and more of the children of the continent are having to grow up without the care of parents and without effective social support systems.

Eonomists at the World Bank estimate that countries with high HIV rates will lose 1 per cent of GDP growth annually. This estimate was supported by Callisto Madavo, Vice President of the World Bank's Africa Region, when he addressed an AIDS conference in Lusaka, Zambia in 1999, saying that HIV was the single great-est threat to future economic development in Africa. Specific reference is made to Kenya, where it is believed that between 1995 and 2005 AIDS will lead to a 14.5 per cent decrease in the country's economic output. If this belief turns out to be true, the poorest nations will suffer even worse economic calamities than those of developing nations.

Female Adolescents and HIV/AIDS

HIV/AIDS is a real danger to the survival of African populations, especially adolescents and in particular female adolescents. The Joint United Nations Programme on HIV/AIDS underscored this when it said that due to unprotected sex, 15,000 people, particularly women, are infected by HIV every day worldwide (Paris, France PANA, 15 March 2000).

HIV/AIDS, an extremely complex disease, has been on the African health scene for about 20 years. In spite of the many resources that have been invested in HIV/AIDS, there is still no known cure. Drugs that are used to prolong life are unaffordable for most Africans, let alone African women. Gestures such as the one by Pfizer, offering to provide Diflucan at no cost to South Africa (*Wall Street Journal*, 4 March 2000) are rare. In Africa, the disease is primarily transmitted heterosexually. The UN warning that one of the world's deadliest diseases is not only taking a toll on women, but also breaking down the institution of extended families and shifting gender roles in third world society (*Gender-AIDS*, 16 March 2000), is powerful and should not be taken lightly by Africans. For reasons given above, Africa ought to intensify efforts to develop effective HIV/AIDS IEC material for adolescents, and in particular females, in order to avoid a collapse of African societies.

According to the *Report on the Global HIV/AIDS Epidemic* (December 1997) there were 16,000 new HIV infections a day globally, of which 90 per cent were in devel-oping countries. 1,600 were from children under 15 years of age. About 14,000 were in adults, of whom over 40 per cent were women and over 50 per cent were aged 15–24 years. In Africa, the adolescent age group of concern stretches up to 35 years. The concern over female adolescents and HIV/AIDS was that there was a general perception that female adolescents were free from HVI/AIDS. This implies

93

that older men tend to get more sexually attracted to female adolescents than to older women. Sexual harassment, which is already being experienced in African communities, becomes one of the means of getting through to these female adolescents when they do not comply with sexual advances. The female adolescents still date male adolescents, creating a vicious circle of HIV/STI transmissions. One of the ways this circle can be broken is by empowering girls and young women with appropriate information on HIV/AIDS and sexual harassment, and creating an environment where they can share experiences and learn of success stories in avoiding HIV/STI transmissions and how to fight sexual harassment.

Some Key HIV/AIDS Challenges Faced by Female Adolescents

Biological Factors Leading to Women's Vulnerability to HIV/AIDS

The mode of transmission of HIV in women in Africa is largely heterosexual, implying that both men and women have equal exposure. According to the March 2000 WHO Fact Sheet, there are biological factors that make women more vulnerable to HIV infections. To begin with, women have larger mucosal surface and microlesions which can occur during intercourse may be entry points for the virus. Young women are even more susceptible to HIV infection in this respect. Second, there is more virus in the sperm than there is in vaginal secretions. Third, women are at least four times more vulnerable to HIV infection than men because of the presence of untreated sexually transmitted infections. Lastly, coerced sex increases the risk of microlesions.

Socio-economic Factors that Make Women Targets of HIV/AIDS

The need for female adolescents to survive economically and the cultural practice of polygamous marriages renders female adolescents open to HIV/STI infections. The notion that female adolescents are free from STI means that adult males are sexually attracted to female adolescents, creating a circle of STI transmissions. The statistics contained in the Report on the Global HIV/AIDS Epidemic are nothing less than traumatising. The staggering figure of 16,000 new HIV infections a day, averaging between 840,000–5,856,000 infections per year spells a severe population depletion in the next century if the spread of HIV/AIDS is not controlled to levels of elimination. Considering the fact that 90 per cent of the infections are in developing countries and the majority of them in Africa, these figures cast a dark cloud over Africa's development and future. The picture is even gloomier when one looks at the number of infections in children under 15 years of age. The future of Africa will be stifled if children do not get a chance to live to adulthood. The 14,000 infections in adults touch on the economically active age group. Of the 40 per cent infections in women, it is the 50 per cent infections in the 15–24 year old age group that are the focus of this paper. The strategy of this paper is to cater for female adolescents aged 15–35 years.

Female Adolescents' Responsibility for Health Care

African female adolescents have responsibilities that go beyond those carried by their mothers. They, like their mothers, bear the psychological and physical burden of AIDS care. Adult African women manage the homes, whereas female adolescents are implementation resources for their families. This means they carry out orders given by their mothers and other elders in the family. From the time they develop from the toddler stage into little girls, they are inducted into the management of female chores. They are taught to cook and clean for the family, draw water and collect fuel-wood for the household, and to take care of siblings and sick members of the family, thereby becoming exposed to communicable diseases. This is evidenced by the AIDS Home-Based Care System in Zambia which shows that the majority of persons who nurse AIDS patients at home are women. The female adolescents find themselves following in the footsteps of the female adults. Until good IEC programmes for home-based care of AIDS patients are developed, the risky of infection among female adolescents is very high.

Problems of Communicating HIV/AIDS Information to Women
HIV/AIDS Policy

The omission of gender concerns in policy documents undermines the status of gender organs as key instruments in health promotion for females. This affects IEC programmes in general and especially IEC for HIV/AIDS. The efforts of international and national institutions and NGOs to reduce HIV infections would be more effective if health policy instruments addressed gender issues in health.

Although individual Heads of State have broken the silence on HIV/AIDS, there is a need to address the issue of IEC policy on HIV/AIDS. The African leaders that have advocated for action against HIV/AIDS are the Ugandan President, Yoweri Museveni, and recently President Olusegun Obasanjo of Nigeria. In Zimbabwe, employers have introduced a levy for HIV/AIDS in an attempt to mitigate the impact of AIDS on their employees. In order to combat HIV/AIDS, governmental, inter-governmental and non-governmental organisations must work together to formulate policies that are aimed at reducing HIV infections. So far there are no known HIV/AIDS policies. On 3 April 2000 Ilse Egers and Joost Hoppenbrouwer sent out a request for HIV/AIDS policies and programmes for employees through a listserv called af-aids@hivnet.ch, but by 7 April 2000, no response had been circulated on the listserv. This may be an indication that nobody cared to respond, or that there are no policies on the subject, or that the respondents answered directly to the inquirers. Whatever the case might be, it would have been interesting to have information on where policies and programmes on HIV/AIDS existed.

IEC for HIV/AIDS Initiatives is Gender Blind

IEC programmes in general do not address gender-specific issues. In the absence of policies or affirmative action plans to address the health of females and empower them to take care of their own health and to make decisions about it, the issue of IEC for HIV/AIDS with a gender bias becomes more difficult. Health organs and institutions do not consider engendering their health education programmes, except on matters of reproductive health. Even though some health ministries, such as the Ministry of Health in Zambia, have gender desks, owing to the Beijing Platform of Action to which they are signatories, it remains to be seen how these relatively new desks will address gender issues on HIV/AIDS.

Access to Communication and Information Technologies for IEC for HIV/AIDS

One of the ways in which the HIV/AIDS in Africa could be reduced is through the dissemination of appropriately packaged HIV/AIDS information using a multi-media format. In implementing IEC programmes for HIV/AIDS, communication problems issues become major issues in an environment where road networks are generally of poor quality, telephone services cover less than 10 per cent of the population, radio and television ownership is a privilege of a few urban residents, computer technology is just beginning to enter the market and where snail mail genuinely merits its name. In particular, communicating HIV/AIDS education information to women, and especially to female adolescents, becomes very difficult. This is due to several factors, one of which is lack of access to radio and television. Even in cases where the technology is available, it is a privilege of men and male adolescents. The technology and its maintenance are above most people's economic means. Transmission capabilities of most public or national broadcasters are poor; telephone links are in most cases limited to urban areas and to the privileged few. The times when HIV/AIDS programmes are transmitted are inappropriate for women and so the list goes on.

Efforts Made to Solve HIV/AIDS IEC Problems

Society of Women and AIDS in Africa (SWAA)

This African region-based NGO draws its membership from organisations with similar aims and objectives. Individual national chapters develop country-specific objectives. The effectiveness of SWAA branches depends on the resourcefulness and vision of the national leadership. Much is attained where the vision and targets are clearly presented and the implementation schedule adhered to. For reasons given earlier regarding constraints faced by NGOs, it is not always possible to get around the problems. It is worthy of mention that SWAA has positive objectives aimed at reducing HIV/AIDS among African women.

Society for Women and AIDS in Zambia (SWAZ)

SWAZ, the Zambian chapter of SWAA, has as one of its main objectives education and communication for HIV/AIDS to the womenfolk. The SWAZ approach to HIV/AIDS education uses the quantitative approach through discussion groups. The target groups are less privileged women striving to earn a living by selling foodstuffs. This group is generally composed of mixed age groups. To reach this group, SWAZ organises lunch hour meetings within the market place to which all marketers are invited. The facilitators at these meetings are members of SWAZ. Marketers are also encouraged to facilitate when they show an ability to do so. The success of this method of educating women on HIV/AIDS is that they participate in the group discussions, thereby giving the facilitators insights into the problems faced by women in trying to avoid HIV infections.

The second target group for HIV/AIDS education is sex workers. This group is largely composed of younger women who are brought together by an NGO called Tasinta (meaning 'we have come to the road's end'). SWAZ collaborates with Tasinta on HIV/AIDS education. Tasinta offices are used for HIV/AIDS education campaigns. The results of this combined HIV/AIDS education is that the sex workers are taught how to engage in protected sex. Most important is that some of them find alternative ways of generating income, and others stop sex work altogether.

Pilot by a Religious Organisation in 2001

A local church group in Zimbabwe is currently developing a proposal entitled HEALTH BY THE WORD. The project targets female adolescents, empowering them to manage their own health and to earn a living. Without using the stigmatised terms HIV and AIDS, the proposal very subtly encourages girls to adhere to Christian morals and become role models in their communities. The project aims at identifying initially ten female adolescents who are willing to stand tall for better management of their health and poverty reduction, while at the same time maintaining a high moral standard in all their dealings. The target audiences for the HEALTH BY THE WORD project are the five nations in the Southern African sub-region that are targeted by Hear the Word Ministries. The concept is based on a snowball effect of impacting the female adolescents in the five nations. Key to the project is that young women and girls give testimonies in various communities about high moral standards.

Possibilities for the Effective Use of IEC to Reduce HIV/AIDS Infection

Rural and Poor Urban Communities as Targets

Female adolescents in rural and urban poor communities receive less information about HIV/AIDS and sexual harassment than other sections of the community, yet they too face the same risks from the two evils. It is for this reason that they should be targeted by IEC on these issues. Community-based organisations are ideal for disseminating HIV/AIDS information. Existing organisations such as schools, health facilities, libraries and other such structures are appropriate as information sources for rural and urban adolescents. Community leaders of all categories are strategically placed to receive and distribute IEC material on HIV/AIDS. Family and community leaders are the first level institutions for HIV/AIDS prevention. School children can become agents for carrying and delivering HIV/AIDS information to families and friends because schools are the most readily available institutions on the African continent. The next most effective institutions to deliver HIV/AIDS education are religious organisations because the are usually widespread in communities. Their impact on HIV/AIDS education is only likely to be effective if they put aside their denominational differences and unite in the fight against the disease. Ideally health institutions should take the lead in HIV/AIDS education; they are to a large degree responsible for designing the IEC material. Gender desks in ministries of health and women's NGOs are responsible for engendering IEC material for HIV/AIDS. Dissemination of HIV/AIDS information to women, and especially to adolescents, should be sensitive to cultural values and norms.

Status of Information Needs of Target Communities

In general, information supply to rural areas and urban poor is inadequate. It is even worse in HIV/AIDS information because of the taboos attached to discussing sex issues in public and the poor state of health information in most of Africa. Female adolescents lose out on HIV/AIDS information for reasons of gender inequality and access to information and technology, which have been discussed earlier. This paper seeks to set out ways of empowering female adolescents to care for their own health, specifically to protect themselves against HIV/AIDS and sexual harassment. The question of how to convey information to female adolescents using multi-media is a priority in the fight against AIDS.

Policy Considerations for IEC for HIV/AIDS Among Female Adolescents

In view of what has been discussed in this paper there are policy implications in two areas. The first is with governments through Ministries of Education, Health and Community Development. It is important to encourage more women to receive as much education as possible as a way of bridging the gender gap in information and access to information and communications technologies. Some African countries have already put in place policy instruments to promote the education of girls. One other strategy that should be followed is the introduction of HIV/AIDS education in schools.

The second policy area is the need for Ministries of Health to aggressively target female adolescents when preparing HIV/AIDS education messages. Ministries of Community Development could consider forming partnerships with Ministries of Health and Education and with community leaders to educate people about HIV/AIDS.

Policy Instruments Needed to Ensure that Women have Equal Access to Information and Community Technology

The policy instruments needed to bridge the gender gap in HIV/AIDS information and access to information and communications technologies are:

- information and communication technology policy itself which should be gender sensitive
- the Implementation Strategy
- the tools for the implementation of the policy.

Affirmative Action to Promote Women's Access to HIV/AIDS Information

As has already been suggested, affirmative action to enable female adolescents to have equal access to HIV/AIDS information and to information and communications technologies should include

- encouraging female adolescents to aim for good education standards
- the enrolment of equal numbers of girls in school
- giving equal employment opportunities and access to information and communication technologies to girls and encouraging them to take leadership roles in the designing of IEC material and in communities.

The Impact of HIV/AIDS on Social and Economic Development and Education

The Impact of AIDS on Economic and Social Development and the Responses

Alan Whiteside

'The burden of HIV and tuberculosis in the Commonwealth is disproportionate and deserves attention by Heads of Government.'

These are the opening words of a leading article in the *British Medical Journal* just prior to the November 1999 Commonwealth Heads of Government meeting in Durban.[1] According to the authors, although Commonwealth countries represent only 29.5 per cent of the global population, they account for 60.5 per cent of cases of HIV and 42.3 per cent of those of tuberculosis. As with all diseases, the burden of HIV is disproportionately higher in the developing rather than developed countries of the Commonwealth (although it is not uniform even here).

The high-income Commonwealth countries have been able to control the epidemic and HIV prevalence is generally low and declining, although in some specific (and usually marginalised) groups rates are stable or even increasing slowly. The availability of new, and very expensive, highly active antiretroviral therapy means mortality rates have fallen. The impact of the disease, which was already small, has declined.

At present the epidemic is centred on Africa and in particular eastern and southern Africa. Indeed, the highest levels of prevalence recorded anywhere in the world are those of southern African Commonwealth countries. In South Africa the 2000 antenatal survey found that 24.5 per cent[2] of pregnant women attending public health facilities were infected; in Swaziland the figure was 34.2 per cent;[3] and in Botswana it was an astonishing 38.6 per cent.[4]

In Caribbean and Pacific countries HIV prevalence is lower and the epidemic has not spread with the speed and severity experienced in Africa. With the exception of Singapore and Malaysia (where HIV infection is generally under control), there is a paucity of good data for the other Asian Commonwealth countries. Indications are that India may have the greatest number of infections of any one country and that HIV is spreading rapidly there. However, even an estimated 4 to 5 million infections are still minor in a population of one billion.

This article is concerned with the impact of AIDS on economic and social development, and the responses. In an organisation as diverse as the Commonwealth, with the range of different current and projected epidemics, it is not possible to talk of one impact. The effects of the epidemic will ultimately be determined by:

- how many people are infected; and

• who they are.

The importance of numbers is obvious; the more people who are infected, the worse the potential impact. The importance of who is infected should be explored further. For every individual and family an infection is a tragedy. However at the national level the reality is that not all people make an equal contribution to, or demands upon, society. The impact of AIDS will depend on who is infected by age, gender, geographic and social location.

In the high- and middle-income countries where the epidemic is contained, the impact will be largely confined to increased demand on the health services. In poorer countries, the scale of the epidemic will, in the first instance, determine the impact. Thus in the Caribbean and Pacific (and Pakistan, Sri Lanka and Bangladesh) where the epidemic is, in World Bank terms, 'concentrated',[5] the impact is felt by those households unfortunate enough to have infected members and by the health service. India is huge and diverse but there are some parts that are undoubtedly experiencing a generalised epidemic. However, early evidence suggests that again the national impact will be quite limited – partly because there are so many people, but also because the country has vast human resources at all levels. This may be one of the main lessons to be learnt when looking for HIV impact beyond the household, health and community levels. Societies with good human resource endowment in terms of education, training and experience may be less vulnerable to the impact of HIV/AIDS.

Africa not only has a generalised epidemic, it also has a shortage of trained and skilled personnel. It is therefore here that the worst impact will be felt. The next part of this article will cover the effect on economic growth, poverty and development – as it is from these three areas that the economic and social impacts will flow. What will be apparent is that there is a great deal that is not known. The reason for this is that AIDS is a new disease and nowhere has it run its course as yet. The impact will take decades or even generations to work through a society.[6]

AIDS and Economic Growth

There have been attempts to model the macroeconomic impact of AIDS, but these are fraught with difficulty. Overviews identify the mechanisms through which the epidemic may affect macroeconomies as a result of the illness and death of productive members, and the diversion of resources from savings (and eventually investment) to care. There have also been attempts to model the economic impact for specific countries,[7] including Tanzania, Cameroon and Zambia. These models show that HIV may well reduce the rate of economic growth and, over a period of 20 years, this may be significant (up to 25 per cent lower than it would otherwise have been). However, in order to make this prediction, projections of both the AIDS epidemic and economic trends have to be combined. Both are difficult to model and combining them compounds the uncertainty. The dire macroeconomic predictions may be balanced by high economic growth rates as in Uganda (7.2 per cent between 1990 and 1996) and Botswana (4.1 per cent over the same period). Furthermore, some models show that if deaths are concentrated in the least productive members of a society, then in pure economic terms the survivors may be better off, with higher per capita incomes.

In recent years, 'as the epidemic has evolved', it has become evident that there may be unexpected and negative effects on economic growth. For example, a private company faced with increased morbidity and mortality in the workforce may terminate the employment of the sick worker and move swiftly to fill vacant posts. Governments facing the same problem will find that posts remain unfilled and that as a result work does not get done. This could lead to lower levels of efficiency and decision-making. In the education sector, students will simply not be taught, which has long-term implications. Service providers such as electricity and transport firms may be hit. The effects are not immediate or dramatic but will lead to a gradual deterioration in the economic environment.

Poverty

The links between poverty and health are increasingly recognised and understood.[8] It is not clear that AIDS is simply a disease of poverty, although poverty undoubtedly helps drive the epidemic. In the early stages, AIDS appears to infect the relatively well-off; they have the disposable incomes that allow them to travel and, in the case of men, purchase sex. Many more poor people become infected and it is likely that as the epidemic evolves they may be proportionately worse affected. However, we are concerned with impact. What is clear is that AIDS increases poverty and may also increase inequality.

AIDS cases are usually disastrous for households. The infected individual will require medical care and possibly special foods, thus increasing demands on household resources. At the same time, if the person is an adult, illness and death reduce household production capacity, resulting in a decline in household income. Thus households are caught in a double trap of needing more resources at the very time when these may be reduced. The one detailed study of the impact of AIDS on households in Anglophone Africa – from Kagera, Tanzania,[9] shows some impacts. Households experiencing an adult death respond by adjustments in household size and reducing their supply of labour to farming, waged employment and non-farm self-employment in the first three months after the death. In addition, there is a decline in per capita growth rates of both income and consumption; medical treatment and funeral costs pose a major financial burden; and female children may be taken out of school. Research in the adjacent Ugandan district of Rakai showed that adult mortality leads to a decline in household economic status.[10]

Part of the survival strategy will be to sell assets, but:

When richer households purchase assets from AIDS-stricken poorer households, the long-term impact may be to accentuate existing inequalities in the distribution of incomes and assets.[11]

It is also clear that the cost of the disease is being shifted onto households. For example, in parts of southern Africa a migrant worker from a rural area on a contract who falls ill will not have his contract renewed nor will he be repatriated. He can no longer access health benefits through his employment and will not have access to the urban health facilities. There may be no service in the vicinity of his rural home and, as a result, the burden of care falls on his family.

Development[12]

Measuring the economic impact of AIDS is difficult due to lack of hard data. There is one international dataset where the effect of the disease is being seen; this is the Human Development Index (HDI), produced by the United Nations Development Programme (UNDP). The UNDP states, 'The purpose of development is to create an enabling environment for people to enjoy long, healthy and creative lives'.[13] The HDI uses three indicators of the most basic human capabilities: leading a long life; being knowledgeable; and enjoying a decent standard of living – arguing that these can be combined to give an index of human development. The loss of life caused by AIDS is reflected in Table 1. The 1996 Human Development Report (HDR) used 1993 life expectancy figures and AIDS was not considered. Since 1997, AIDS has been taken into account (but not consistently). The disease will also increase infant and child mortality rates, but as yet this is not seen in official data, although models suggest in the worst case that the rates could double.

Table 1. Life expectancy and place in the Human Development Index[14]

| | 1996 | | 1997 | | 1998 | | 1999 | | 2000 | |
	Life Expect.	Rank	Life Expect.	Rank	Life Expect.	Rank	Life Expect.	Rank	Life Expect.	Rank
Botswana	65.2	71	52.3	97	51.7	97	47.4	122	46.2	122
South Africa	63.2	100	63.7	90	64.1	89	54.7	101	53.2	103
Swaziland	57.8	110	58.3	114	58.8	115	60.2	113	60.7	112
Namibia	59.1	116	55.9	118	55.8	107	52.4	115	50.1	115
Zimbabwe	53.4	124	49.0	129	48.9	130	44.1	130	43.5	130
Kenya	55.5	128	53.6	134	53.8	137	52	136	51.3	138
Zambia	48.5	136	42.6	143	42.7	146	40.1	151	40.5	153
Malawi	45.5	157	41.1	161	41.0	161	39.3	159	39.5	163

The effect of HIV and AIDS on development indicators means that development goals need to be re-assessed. This must be done at both national and international levels. For example the OECD[15] set targets that included:

- a reduction by one-half in the proportion of people living in extreme poverty by 2015;

- universal primary education in all countries by 2015;

- demonstrated progress towards gender equality and the empowerment of women by eliminating disparity in primary and secondary education by 2005;

- a reduction by two-thirds in the mortality rates for infants and children under the age of 5 and a reduction by three-quarters in maternal mortality, all by 2015;

- access through the primary health care system to reproductive health services for all individuals of appropriate ages as soon as possible and no later than the year 2015.

However, it is clear that in many countries such targets have become unattainable and need to be reassessed.

Of particular concern is the level of orphaning. Africa's population is young and changes in population structure where adults are lost will result in large numbers of orphans. These children will grow up with less adult attention than might otherwise have been the case. There are increasing numbers of street children and a small (about 5 per cent), but significant, number of 'child-headed' households in Tanzania, Uganda and, no doubt, in other heavily-affected areas. These children have no adult guidance. This will no doubt represent a major and broader impact on 'social capital' in the form of lack of social skills, knowledge, unclear expectations, as well as on detectable and quantifiable declines in levels of formal education.

Responses

What of the responses to the impact of the epidemic? Almost without exception they have been totally inadequate. They have been particularly inadequate at the international and national levels. At the local level non-governmental organisations, community groups and churches have begun to respond. However, these are local responses to a much larger problem and can only meet part of the need. Private companies have begun to respond – but they respond to minimise their exposure, and this may not be in the interests of the nation or their employees.

National governments and development agencies seem totally blasé as to what HIV/AIDS will mean. The exceptions are those concerned with health (government ministries and departments in development agencies). However, they often do not have the breadth of vision or the power to push the multisectoral responses that are needed (and generally they are not listened to anyway). AIDS is beginning to get the profile it deserves – the UN Security Council, at its meeting in January 2000, was indicative of this. However, there is still no real appreciation of the long-term impacts HIV/AIDS will have, or how to respond – and, just as important, how to prioritise the responses.

Conclusion

The impact of HIV/AIDS can be summarised as being long-term, complex and surprising. It will result in growing misery and poverty for many millions of people. At worst it will roll back many of the gains in human development of the past four decades. The issue is primarily a problem for the poorer countries of the world. It may not, therefore, remain on the global agenda, even though the impact is set to get very much worse. AIDS is probably the biggest development challenge for the first quarter of the new century. Getting our response to AIDS right will involve addressing many of the other issues that bedevil the poor of the Commonwealth. I am not optimistic.

Notes

1. Nicoll, A and Godfrey-Fawcett, P (1999). 'HIV and tuberculosis in the Commonwealth', *British Medical Journal* 319: 1086.

2. Department of Health, Republic of South Africa (2000). *National HIV and Syphilis Sero-prevalence Survey of Women Attending Public Antenatal Clinics in South Africa.*

3. Ministry of Health and Social Welfare (2000). *The Kingdom of Swaziland 7th HIV Sentinel Sero-surveillance Report Year 2000.* Swaziland National AIDS/STDs Program, Mbabane, Swaziland.

4. AIDS/STD Unit (2000). *Botswana 2000 HIV Sero-prevalence Sentinel Survey Amongst Pregnant Women and Men with Sexually Transmitted Diseases: A Technical Report.*

5. The World Bank identifies three epidemic stages. Nascent: HIV is less than 5 per cent in all known sub-populations presumed to practise high-risk behaviour for which information is available. Concentrated: HIV prevalence is above 5 per cent in one or more sub-populations presumed to practise high-risk behaviour, but among women attending urban antenatal clinics it is still below 5 per cent. Finally Generalised: HIV has spread far beyond the original sub-population with high-risk behaviour, which are now heavily infected. Prevalence among women attending urban antenatal clinics is 5 per cent or more. The World Bank (1997). *Confronting AIDS Public Priorities in a Global Epidemic.* New York: Oxford University Press, p. 87.

6. The concepts of impact and the time scale are discussed in Barnett, Tony and Whiteside, Alan (2000). 'Guidelines for Preparation and Execution of Studies of the Social and Economic Impact of HIV/AIDS'. UNAIDS.

7. See for example Cuddington, IT (1992). 'Modelling the macro-economic effects of

AIDS, with an application to Tanzania', *World Bank Economic Review* 7, pp. 403–17; Forgy, L and Mwanza, A (1994). 'The Economic Impact of AIDS in Zambia', Lusaka: Ministry of Health; Kambou, G, Devarajan, S and Over, M (1992). 'The economic impact of AIDS in an African country: simulations with a computable general equilibrium model of Cameroon', *Journal of African Economics* 1, pp. 109–30.

8. This is discussed in a number of recent publications, see for example World Health Organisation Department of Health in Sustainable Development, 'Health in Poverty Reduction, Collected Papers', mimeo (undated) and Department for International Development International Development Target Strategy Paper, Consultation Document, 'Better Health for Poor People', DFID, London, November 1999.

9. This is reviewed in Barnett, Tony and Whiteside, Alan with Desmond, Chris (2000). 'The Social and Economic Impact of HIV/AIDS in Poor Countries: a review of studies and lessons'. UNAIDS.

10. Menon, R, Wawer, M, Konde-Lule, J et al (1998). 'The economic impact of adult mortality on households in Rakai District, Uganda', in Ainsworth, M, Fransen, L and Over, M (eds). 'Confronting AIDS: Evidence from the developing world', selected background papers for the World Bank Policy Research Report, *Confronting AIDS: Public Priorities in a global epidemic*. Luxembourg: European Commission and World Bank.

11. de Vlyder, Stefan (1999). 'Issue Paper on Socio-economic Causes and Consequences of HIV/AIDS'. Stockholm: SIDA Health Division Document, 3.

12. For a full discussion of the development impact of AIDS see Barnett, Tony and Whiteside, Alan. 'HIV/AIDS in Africa: Implications for "development" and policy'. Paper presented at the Standing Committee on University Studies of Africa, Fourth SCUSA Inter-university Colloquium, 5–8 September 1999.

13. UNDP (1999). 'Human Development Report 1999'. New York: Oxford University Press, p. 1.

14. United Nations (1996, 1997, 1998, 1999, 2000). 'Human Development Reports'. New York: Oxford University Press. (Note that the life expectancies used for calculating the human development index are for 1993, 1994, 1995 and 1997 respectively.)

15. OECD, 'New Strategies for the Challenges Ahead: A Changing Development Co-operation'. http:www.oecd.org/dac/htm/stc/intro.htm

A Population, Development, Sexual and Reproductive Health Perspective

International Planned Parenthood Federation (IPPF)

Introduction

In the areas hit hardest by the HIV/AIDS pandemic, there is no part of society left unaffected by the disease in some way. AIDS affects every country in the world, but the epidemic has become the greatest threat to development in much of sub-Saharan Africa. Estimates show that 14.5 million people in Commonwealth sub-Saharan Africa alone are affected by HIV with the accompanying devastating impact on the social and economic development of the countries concerned.

AIDS today is no longer simply a public health issue; it cuts across sectors and national boundaries. When we talk of AIDS, we are not talking only about health, but about agriculture, education, the economy. AIDS is indeed at the heart of the development agenda.

The Facts

- 34.3 million in the world are currently living with HIV and some 18.8 million people have died since the beginning of the HIV/AIDS epidemic.

- 3.8 million of them are children and 7.7 million are women; there are 13.2 million AIDS orphans.

- 95 per cent of the people infected with HIV live in developing countries with little access to health services and education.

- Commonwealth countries represent approximately 29 per cent of the world's population, but a figure as high as 60 per cent of global AIDS infections.

- 23.3 million people infected with HIV or living with AIDS are in Africa.

- Latin America and the Caribbean have around 1.7 million people living with HIV infection, of whom nearly 30,000 are children.

- Asia has 6.5 million people living with AIDS and in Eastern Europe people living with HIV rose by a third throughout 1999, reaching a total of 360,000.

Situation Analysis

A World Bank Study in Tanzania has estimated that by the year 2010 AIDS will kill almost 15,000 teachers and 27,000 by the year 2020. The cost of training new teachers could be as high as US$37.8 million. In Malawi, the epidemic has reached crisis proportions. The cost of caring for AIDS patients until they die is estimated to be between US$200–900 (almost four times the country's annual per capita income).

The AIDS epidemic is developing differently from country to country and region to region, depending on local practices, customs and resources available, including the level of knowledge and awareness.

HIV has been a latecomer in Asia with no countries experiencing a major epidemic in the 1980s. However, today HIV/AIDS is a major menace to India, which was once seen as relatively immune to the virus. The UN estimates that HIV/AIDS could cost India $11 billion in health care by 2000.

The epidemic will wipe out all the hard-won gains in life expectancy, maternal and child mortality if we do not expand our resources. Life expectancy at birth in South Africa has dropped dramatically. The same trend is true for other Commonwealth countries such as Botswana, Malawi and Tanzania.

The Response

A Population, Development, Sexual and Reproductive Health Perspective

Despite the bleak picture, much can be done to turn the tide of this disease. Working at the national and local level through Family Planning Associations, IPPF has gathered experience worldwide; growing evidence suggests that AIDS infection can be reduced when programmes are focused and have strong political support, community participation and cross-sectoral partnerships.

The IPPF links national Family Planning Associations in more than 150 countries worldwide. These Associations provide a variety of reproductive health services, including counselling, information and a choice of family planning methods. The FPAs in 53 Commonwealth countries are engaged in a number of activities addressing HIV/AIDS ranging from raising awareness and providing education to prevention and care.

Key Approaches and Strategies

Awareness and Condom Promotion

At the local FPA level there is good experience in condom promotion and local NGOs often have systems in place for logistics and distribution.

For example:

• In India the FPA has embarked on an awareness training campaign targeting

HIV-positive individuals and their families so that they can regain status in their communities;

• The Papua New Guinea Family Planning Association has introduced a condom mail order and inquiry service which has proved very effective since its introduction.

Clinical and Community-based Services

Many FPAs have the relevant infrastructures in place, which can be strengthened to help people who suffer or fear an sexually transmitted infection, including HIV.

For example:

• The Family Planning Association in Mozambique provides assistance and counselling to HIV/AIDS carriers and patients at home and in the community.

Reaching Women

It has been increasingly recognised that there is a need for a special focus on women who, often due to culturally determined gender roles, are left with little control over their own sexuality – making them particularly vulnerable to HIV. Family planning programmes are often the only contact women in developing countries have with organised health programmes.

Reaching Young People

At the grassroots level, FPAs work closely with young people who are particularly vulnerable to STI and now to HIV infection.

For example:

• The 'Youth for Youth' projects in Ghana, Botswana and Sierra Leone aim to test and develop an effective participatory model to enable young adults to protect themselves against unwanted pregnancies, sexually transmitted diseases (STDs), including HIV/AIDS, and unsafe abortions. Key to the innovative approach of this project is the provision of information, education, counselling and services to young people, and the participation of young adults employed as peer-educators and community-based distributors of condoms to both in and out of school youth.

Male Involvement

Men are a crucial audience for STI/HIV/AIDS prevention. Projects run by the local Family Planning Associations in Ghana and Kenya have shown excellent results. These projects aim at enlisting the support of men in the reproductive lives of their wives or female partners and also at encouraging them to use condoms for prevention of STI/HIV/AIDS.

For example:

- In Kenya, three 'male only' clinics were established on a pilot basis. These clinics offer a range of reproductive and sexual health services, including vasectomy, treatment of reproductive track infections and advice on AIDS prevention. Evaluation results show the positive impact in changing men's attitude and behaviour. Men are now enlisted as motivators in the prevention of HIV/AIDS.

Quality Care

Many FPAs provide high quality care and have the confidence of clients – particularly women – for discussing problems related to sexual reproductive health. They offer privacy and therefore can help alleviate the fear of stigmatisation among women who go for a consultation for a reproductive tract infection or because they fear HIV infection.

Education

FPAs have developed educational materials and undertaken information and educational activities both in service delivery facilities as well as in the communities.

For example:

- The FPA in the Dominican Republic runs a project on communication for behavioural change in STI/HIV/AIDS and sexual reproductive health education, targeting youth peer educators. Information, education and communication materials are produced and educational activities for parents, teachers and community leaders are held, combined with condom distribution. In addition, the project has included training and a monitoring plan for staff members of governmental bodies, NGOs and the National Youth Network for AIDS prevention efforts.

- In the Solomon Islands, the FPA offers Family Life Education which includes AIDS education through radio, reaching 90 per cent of the population.

Collaboration and Commitments

Collaboration across sectors with key stakeholders is as crucial for HIV/AIDS efforts as are commitments – at the local, national and international level.

International Commitment

The international community held a number of key global conferences in the 1990s which set out programmes of actions to address population, development, sexual and reproductive health, women's empowerment, gender equity and equality, as well as poverty. These included the International Conference on Population and Development (ICPD), Cairo 1994; the Fourth World Women's Conference, Beijing 1995; and the World Social Summit, Copenhagen, 1995. At each of the conferences governments made commitments and pledges to address key issues in these fields, including HIV/AIDS, which were strengthened most recently at the five-year reviews of the implementation of these promises.

At the five-year review of the Cairo Conference – known as Cairo + 5 – governments addressed the increasingly urgent issue of HIV/AIDS. The final UN Document adopted by the UN General Assembly includes calls for governments to ensure that provision of, and services for, STIs and HIV/AIDS are an integral component of reproductive and sexual health programmes at the primary health care level.

Gender, aged-based and other differences in individuals' vulnerability to HIV infection should be addressed in prevention and education programmes and services; governments are urged to ensure that by 2005 at least 90 per cent of young men and women aged 15–24 have access to the information, education and services necessary to develop the life skills required to reduce their vulnerability to HIV infection.

At the five-year review of the Beijing Women's Conference, held in 2000, there was increasing emphasis on tackling the HIV/AIDS pandemic, with calls for the global community to increase its efforts. Provisions relating to women and health include putting strong emphasis on the gender aspects of HIV/AIDS and STIs – pointing out their disproportionate impact on women's and girls' health and calling for proper polices and measures to address these challenges. The Beijing review also explicitly addressed the situation of the girl child affected by HIV/AIDS – as an infected person, care provider or orphan.

Political Commitment

If progress is to be made in the fight against HIV/AIDS, the strong commitment of governments is clearly necessary. As witnessed at the 1999 Commonwealth Heads of Government Meeting (CHOGM) in Durban, Heads of State have made personal and political commitments to tackling the epidemic. Such commitments are key pledges to follow-up on and expand.

In October 1999, the President of Kenya, Arap Moi, who until then had given the epidemic only a passing mention, at last declared AIDS a 'national disaster'. The Kenyan government has now decided to allow AIDS awareness to be taught in schools. As stated by a Masogo nurse, 'Schools are very near . . . It is the health centres that are far away'. This emphasis is important as the most recent UN statistics predict that across Kenya half of the girls who turn 15 this year will be infected with the virus during their lifetimes.

Uganda was ravaged by the disease in the early 1990s. It was one of the first countries to launch an aggressive public education campaign. The campaign was led by President Yoweri Musevini, who solicited foreign donors to support the effort. By the late 1990s, Uganda was the first African nation where the rate of new infection had declined and has thus become a model for the continent.

Key Future Actions: Working in Partnerships

HIV/AIDS is a health and human tragedy. As the urgency to address the issues grows, key actions – based on active partnerships – must be identified. Key actions include:

- Recognition of the prevention of HIV/AIDS as a national duty;

- Governments, in partnership with all stakeholders, must activate plans and commit resources for the reduction of the spread of the virus through prevention;

- A multi-disciplinary approach is needed involving expertise and experience in communications, the media, community development, sexuality and health behaviour;

- All programmes must be gender-sensitive and respectful of cultural values and human rights;

- Training must be provided for a range of carers, workers and others involved at all levels;

- Dual protection – the prevention of both STI/HIV/AIDS infection and unwanted pregnancy through the use of a condom and/or other contraceptive method – must be promoted;

- Young people, who are particularly vulnerable to STI/HIV/AIDS, must be addressed specifically.

The task is large, yet achievable if we work in close partnerships, across sectors, and with a commitment matched by action.

For further information visit IPPF's website: www.ippf.org

Acknowledgement

This material was originally presented at the conference, 'The HIV/AIDS Crisis: A Commonwealth Response', Marlborough House, London, 7 December 2000.

AIDS in Africa: The Urban Environment

Ian Douglas, David Hall and John Anderson

Introduction

Towns and cities in Africa are growing faster than most other urban areas. The 1990–95 annual growth rates of Maputo and Yaoundé were 7.6 and 6.6 per cent. Lagos grew from 0.29 million people in 1950 to 10.3 million in 1995 and is expected to reach 24.6 million by 2015. Only Mumbai (Bombay) and Tokyo are forecast to exceed Lagos in population by 2015. Only Qingdao in China had as fast a growth rate as Maputo. Much of the urban growth comes from in-migration of poor people from rural areas and smaller towns. The urban livelihoods of most recent migrants, and of many of the poorest long established urban families, are insecure. An estimated 75 per cent of urban employment in many sub-Saharan African countries is in informal jobs (World Bank, 1995).

African urban areas generally have fewer homes connected to water supplies, sewerage and electricity than towns and cities in other continents. While Banjul, Lilongwe, Maputo, Dar-es-Salaam, Kampala and Lusaka all have less than 40 per cent of their households connected to the water supply, Havana, Dhaka, Manila, Hanoi, Bogota, Rio de Janeiro and Quito all have 80 per cent or more connected. Sewerage is available to less than 10 per cent of households in cities like Douala, Yaounde, Maseru, Ibadan, Lagos, Dar-es-Salaam and Kampala. Such problems make urban living conditions unhealthy for many people. In Accra, 18 per cent of all deaths are caused by infections (largely diarrheal diseases, malaria and measles). Part of this high percentage is due to the large number under-five-year-olds in the population, indicating that infant mortality is high, a condition taken by health statisticians to indicate poor living conditions.

Great differences in living conditions and health occur in African urban areas. Social status greatly affects vulnerability to disease. While the general urban population may often be healthier than the general rural population, those living in urban slums and squatter settlements often are much less healthy than the general rural population.

Women and children are particularly vulnerable. Poor children in towns and cities are exposed to a host of toxic and infectious substances and agents during their daily activities, play, schooling and eating. Lack of sanitation and the use of contaminated water lead to severe diarrhea and other intestinal disorders. Most of the 5 million children estimated to die from diarrheal diseases every year in the developing world are from poor urban families. Respiratory infections, the second most prominent cause of death among children in the developing world, are particularly associated with urban overcrowding, and indoor and outdoor air pollution.

116

Ill health among poor urban children is often the product of the interplay of malnutrition, lack of sanitation, exposure to infectious diseases and toxic pollutants, as well as lack of access to health care. Social factors also affect the health of young urban people and urban women.

Urban women also face increased health risks in towns and cites, again as a result of social factors. Women use smoky stoves in inadequately ventilated, poorly constructed, cramped homes and often have to collect and use the contaminated water. Cooking on wood, charcoal and paraffin, abundant dust mites, ants, flies and cockroaches, and proximity within dwellings to smokers particularly influence child health. Women take care of the sick children and pick up infections from them and are particularly at risk during pregnancy

Violence is often a significant cause of death among adolescent males in rapidly growing cities. Thus, for many people, the urban environment is unhealthy and increases their vulnerability to disease. Superimposed on this general vulnerability are all the factors that contribute to the spread of HIV/AIDS.

HIV/AIDS Issues in the Sector

In a world where 15,000 people a day catch AIDS, sub-Saharan Africa is now home to 70 per cent of all HIV-infected individuals; of all AIDS deaths, 80 per cent have occurred in this region alone. Ninety per cent of all children with perinatal infection and 95 per cent of all AIDS orphans reside in sub-Saharan Africa, despite the fact that it contains only 10 per cent of the world's population. The sheer number of Africans infected by this epidemic is overwhelming. Currently, an estimated 34 million people living in sub-Saharan Africa have been infected with the virus, 11.5 million (a quarter of them children) have died. In 1998 AIDS was responsible for an estimated two million African deaths or 5,500 funerals per day. Despite the scale of death, there are more Africans living with HIV than ever before: 21.5 million adults and one million children. In Botswana, Namibia, Swaziland and Zimbabwe, current estimates show that 20–30 per cent of people aged 15 to 49 are living with HIV. In Zimbabwe, 30–50 per cent of all pregnant women are now infected, and at least one-third of these women will pass the infection on to their babies. South Africa, which escaped much of the epidemic in the 1980s, is now being particularly hard hit; one in seven new infections on the African continent is occurring in South Africa. Perhaps more alarming is the recent test of youths in Sundumbili township in KwaZulu-Natal where 80 per cent were HIV-positive. This can be projected into an implied death rate of 80 per cent of young people before they reach the age of 30. Already communities and nations are facing massive losses of people in youth and middle age.

Within each country the HIV epidemic has developed in a different manner among various communities and social groups. In the early stages of the epidemic, urban people and rural communities along main roads were most rapidly affected.

Urban centres and market towns still tend to have a substantially higher occurrence of HIV than rural areas, but this is by no means always the case. Civil conflict, forced movements of people and intense migration greatly influence the spread of HIV. In some rural areas of Kenya, Uganda and Tanzania, HIV rates are similar to those of nearby towns.

In West Africa, some 1.7 million people leave the country for the city each year (David, 1997). Many workers are involved in a seasonal circular migration, to areas of work for several months and then back to their home communities. Such 'commuting' can be either local or international and is often made up of travelling populations such as traders or long-distance truck drivers whose mobility and patterns of recreational activity make them a high-risk group for AIDS.

Urban poverty creates particularly difficult circumstances for many women. Weak economies and high rates of unemployment have led many women to sell sexual services which are often seen as the only means of survival available to them. In some countries, female clerks are an example of the type of worker who can survive only by occasionally selling sex in exchange for the protection and gifts higher-ranking men can offer them. Female students without family support often engage in a type of informal prostitution to support themselves during their studies.

Prostitution in the urban environment takes varying forms. Two categories of prostitute have been described in Ghana, based on how they reach their clients. 'Seaters' are well-organised professionals working in the most affluent parts of cities and have their own aid agencies. 'Roamers' tend to be younger and more enterprising, contacting their clients in bars, hotels and on the street; this prostitution constitutes only a temporary alternative means of economic survival, which means that they have weak group cohesion and are difficult to reach during AIDS prevention campaigns (David, 1997). Prostitution and its role in HIV/AIDS diffusion are thus major features of the urban environment and intimately related to urban poverty and the struggles poor women face for survival.

The impact of HIV/AIDS on the urban health sector is heavily taxing the already overstretched medical services. HIV-related patients occupy 39 per cent of the beds in the Kenyatta National Hospital in Nairobi, Kenya. Tuberculosis has become the leading cause of death among people with HIV infection because HIV weakens people's immune systems. Sickness and death due to AIDS is growing rapidly among health care personnel, but as yet few countries have as yet fully understood the epidemic's impact on human resources in the health sector. A study in Zambia showed that in one hospital, deaths among health care workers increased 13-fold between 1980 and 1990, largely because of HIV. Rising rates of HIV infection in health-care workers will increase rates of absenteeism, reduce productivity, and lead to increased costs of death benefits, staff recruitment and training of new personnel.

Clearly HIV/AIDS has implications for the whole of urban society. Many of the

issues are related to urban infrastructure and access to health service
appropriate medicines. Dealing with the problem requires both spe
programmes and the integration of prevention and care packages
urban environmental programmes. Development agencies need to inɔiuue AIDS
in their urban programmes and community action plans. National family planning
programmes with 'teaching clinics' can have a beneficial impact. Successful programmes involve multisectoral and multilevel partnerships between government
departments and between government and civil society, with AIDS being routinely
factored into individual and joint agendas. Authorities appear to shy away from
publishing the worst statistics, assuming that the epidemic will die down of its own
accord.

Addressing the Issue

In many ways, the HIV/AIDS epidemic is an outcome of the social and economic
changes that have led to rapid urbanisation and the crowding of people into poor
quality urban environments. Transmission is, in part, related to patterns of work,
travel, housing and poverty. Thus an integrated approach to HIV/AIDS is closely
related in concept to a holistic view of improving communities and the living
environment in human settlements. Key interlinked targets must be poverty alleviation, improved water and sanitation, job creation, better housing and greater
social cohesion. These are all targets of the United Nations Habitat Agenda whose
implementation in the Commonwealth is being advocated and encouraged by the
Commonwealth Consultative Group on Human Settlements through a partnership between the Commonwealth Secretariat and the Commonwealth Human
Ecology Council. The benefits for alleviation of the epidemiological conditions
that foster the HIV/AIDS epidemic and for society as a whole, of programmes
directed at urban environmental issues need to be brought to the fore. Infrastructure improvements have to be interlinked with building and strengthening
community ties and cohesion and with planned contraception programmes within
general health improvements. Progress has to be monitored and reported to ensure
that initiatives are maintained and have continuing effectiveness. Initiatives such
as the preparation of Community Sustainable Development Indicators and
Community Learning, Information and Communications Centres can assist in this
process and can widen to advance appropriate health improvement issues.

Commonwealth Collaborative Action

- Implement the Habitat Agenda and, in particular, follow up the suggestion
  made by members of the Commonwealth Consultative Group on Human
  Settlements in Durban in 1999 that there should be a Habitat Agenda for
  Africa;

- Develop an integrated, holistic, ecological approach to strengthening communities through greater security of tenure and jobs, and through education with an understanding of 'safer sex';

- Develop and implement national policies on urban settlements and family planning;

- Encourage capacity building at local government level for integrated planning of urban settlements, community development and health improvement;

- Strengthen local NGOs so that they work closely with communities to enhance partnerships with the public and private sectors on projects ranging from the enhancement of housing, water and sanitation, and employment and environmental conditions to public health improvement and social development;

- Develop existing Commonwealth Secretariat-Foundation-Professional Organisation-NGO partnerships concerned with human settlements to embrace health improvement issues in the urban context, with special emphasis on HIV/AIDS.

Acknowledgement

This material was originally presented at the conference, 'The HIV/AIDS Crisis: A Commonwealth Response', Marlborough House, London, 7 December 2000.

References available on request.

Mitigating the Impact of HIV/AIDS on Education Systems in Southern Africa

Carol Coombe

The gains of *Education for All, 1990–2000* (EFA) are being undone by the AIDS pandemic, particularly in southern Africa. Nevertheless, most countries in the region, as elsewhere, do not yet factor the influence of AIDS into education planning. While attention has been given by many ministries to teaching children about safe sex through the Life Skills curriculum, little has as yet been done to assess the actual and potential damage of AIDS to learning, to the teaching service and to the education system itself.

What must be done to stop HIV/AIDS from undermining the foundations of quality education for all? What can be done to mitigate the pandemic's consequences? Does education's planning and management paradigm need to change? This brief article addresses the first question, in an attempt to find practical answers to the other two.

The Threat of AIDS to Education Systems

Education systems in southern Africa are vulnerable to AIDS because of political, economic and social instability. They are characterised by high attrition, repetition and drop-out rates, and over-age enrolments. Increasing viral transmission further compounds these inefficiencies. Large numbers of traumatised and deprived AIDS orphans live outside community control and are lost to schooling. Rising STD (Sexually Transmitted Disease) infections among scholars and teachers make them more vulnerable to HIV, while old killers like tuberculosis, malaria and cholera take advantage of their depleted immune systems. Morbidity and mortality rates among learners and educators are rising inexorably. In southern Africa, life expectancy after HIV infection is 6–8 years.

Information about AIDS in southern Africa demands universal attention:

- In southern Africa, life expectancy rose from 44 in the 1950s to 59 in the 1990s, but will fall to 45 by 2010. Twenty per cent of 15–19 year olds are HIV-positive. At least 10 per cent of school children are infected.

- In Mozambique, there will be more than 250,000 AIDS orphans by the end of 2000, and one-quarter of all children will be living in a family where HIV is present.

- In Namibia, school enrolments in 2010 will be at least 8 per cent lower than in 1998. About 3,500 serving teachers will die by 2010. AIDS-related teacher attrition is likely to be about 3 per cent per annum over ten years.

- In South Africa, at least 12 per cent of teachers are HIV-positive. It has been estimated that in the coming years, more than 50 per cent of 15-year-olds will die of AIDS or AIDS-related illness. Prevalence in girls aged 15–19 has risen from 12.7 per cent to 21 per cent in 1999.

- In Swaziland, about one in five Swazis over 14 are HIV-positive. The population is already 7 per cent below expected levels, and by 2016 it will be 42 per cent lower than projected without AIDS. There are currently 35,000 AIDS orphans; by 2016, there may be 120,000.

- In Zambia mortality among educators in 1998 was 70 per cent higher than that of the 15–49 age group, and equalled two-thirds of annual Teaching Training College output. By 2005 losses will exceed Teacher Training College output. In 2010, there will be 1,660,000 AIDS orphans, and 7 per cent of Zambia's households will be child-headed, without adults.

The Impact of AIDS

As a result of morbidity and mortality of this magnitude, AIDS is already having a significant impact on education in the region.

Fewer children enrol in school because:

- HIV-positive mothers die young, with fewer progeny;

- children die young of AIDS complications;

- children who are ill, impoverished, orphaned or carers for younger children, or those who are earners or producers, are out of school.

Qualified Teachers and Officials are Being Lost to Education

Teachers and officials are particularly vulnerable to infection because of their comparatively high incomes, often remote postings and social mobility. Other teachers are being lost as they leave education for better jobs elsewhere. The capacity of colleges and faculties of education to keep up with educator attrition will be undermined by their own staff losses. There will be fewer tertiary students as secondary school output and quality goes down, and as higher education itself declines due to staff attrition.

In some Southern Africa Development Community (SADC) countries, education management, administration systems and procedures, and financial control are already deteriorating. Under such circumstances, ministries will find it difficult to provide formal education of the scope and quality envisioned after Jomtien. Sickness and death benefit costs are rising, along with additional costs for teacher training. Governments are under increasing pressure to finance other social sectors.

Contributions from parents and communities are declining, and many households are no longer willing or able to keep children in school. Thus the cost of schooling is shifting back to governments.

What is incalculable is the trauma which threatens to overwhelm children, teachers, parents and their schools. At the very least, in pragmatic rather than humanitarian terms, school effectiveness must be expected to decline when as many as 30–40 per cent of teachers, officials and children are ill, lacking morale, and unable to concentrate on learning, teaching and professional matters.

All of this means that education ministries must anticipate a real reversal of development gains, that further development will be more difficult and that current development goals will be unattainable.

Mitigating the Consequences of HIV/AIDS on Education Systems

One international education specialist has concluded that:

We education sector people seem to be completely at a loss as to what to do next for the education sector. The situation is desperate and getting worse. This is not merely a health problem, but a major social problem, particularly for education systems. The extent and the nature of the problem for the education sector is not known or is inadequately known. There is no apparent contingency plan for the education sector. These are frightening conclusions that need to be widely understood by the education community.

There are things that can be done. It requires that educators – all of those in and out of government who are responsible for the well-being of the education sector – recognise the problem, and then think, plan and manage more systematically.

1. Strengthening the Foundation for Counteracting AIDS
- **Collecting information.** We need more and better information. How can it be collected systematically? Who is responsible for regular reporting, collecting and collating? Who will analyse it and feed it into the decision-making process?

- **Developing consensus.** It should be possible to reach agreement within the education sector, through consultation among all partners, about how to protect the quality of education. Consensus needs to take account of, and perhaps be driven by, local practitioners. This consensus should be reflected in a policy and regulatory framework which promotes learning about AIDS in classrooms, protects the legal and constitutional rights of learners and educators affected by AIDS, and provides a conceptual framework for taking action to protect education quality.

- **Policy and planning.** Consultative structures and systems are required which will allow ministries of education, singly and in concert with others in each region, to plan responses to the AIDS pandemic.

- **Creating management capacity.** Ministries of education are at least under a moral obligation to deploy the best managers and leaders to counteract the pandemic. Because so much is at stake, it is essential to recruit and appoint, at national and local levels, dedicated teams of proven, mature senior managers, on contract if necessary. This is not a part-time assignment for individuals dotted around the bureaucracy. Fighting AIDS, protecting children, teachers and other educators, and the system itself, is a full-time assignment, at least in the short- to medium-term, until the situation stabilises. Staff job descriptions, and unit mandates and job descriptions, must be completely transparent and clearly defined.

- **Mobilising resources.** Money is not flowing adequately to local administrations and NGOs who bear much responsibility for supporting, advising and caring in schools and communities. Teachers and principals are often left without adequate resources to respond to children and colleagues in crisis. NGOs, community-based organisations (CBOs), traditional leaders and faith-based organisations do not generally receive adequate recognition or compensation for the vital role they are playing in concert with government in combating and mitigating this pandemic.

Co-operation and trust need to characterise the education sector's response to AIDS. That means, for example:

- breaking the impasse between politicians, government officials, NGOs and institutional activists, academics, and the media, which too often inhibits swift and tangible assistance to children, teachers and the system itself;

- nominating the school as the ultimate CBO, the centre for local response, working with grassroots organisations, local practitioners and activists, parents and district officials, teachers and business leaders;

- creating working linkages with regions, among provinces and districts;

- listening to what teachers and district officials have to say about what needs to be done, how it can be done and what resources they need to do it;

- depending more on teachers' unions to get the AIDS message out to their members.

Four strong structures already exist to carry messages to people throughout South Africa: schools, unions, traditional authorities and faith-based organisations. Their potential for leadership on AIDS issues at local levels requires further exploration and elaboration.

2. Understanding the Impact of the Pandemic
It is possible to take swift action on the basis of what is now known about AIDS from observation and existing research evidence. It is true, nevertheless, that much more systematic quantitative information is needed about:

- the demographic implications of the pandemic for education;

- the numbers of people likely to fall ill, the duration of illness and age distribution;

- the numbers of people dying, analysed by age;

- the pandemic's impact on population size and distribution;

- teacher and child illness, death and attrition rates so as to project teacher requirements, enrolment shifts, geographical and age shifts, etc.;

- regional, cultural and socio-economic differences, and what problems these might pose.

Data, survey and testing results, research conclusions and analyses do not need to be perfect. Headway can be made using available information, as long as it is collated and made accessible to planners and managers. Existing school and district reporting forms can provide much information on attrition, repetition, illness and dropouts, and planners and analysts can extrapolate from them without adding unnecessarily to schools' reporting burdens.

Concerns about the quality of education provision require more detailed research and analysis. Some difficult matters raised during the course of a recent survey in South Africa include:

- How do existing knowledge, beliefs and value systems complicate Life Skills teaching, and its integration in the core curriculum?

- How can the content of schooling be adapted to the pandemic so that children learn what they need to learn in terms of essential literacy and numeracy, Life Skills and values related to AIDS, work-oriented skills, social and coping skills?

- What should the education system look like in future, that is, what needs to be done to ensure that it:

  - provides more comprehensive, integrated care for young children in distress and those who look after them;

  - ensures that AIDS-affected children get into and continue in school, or are offered alternative basic education programmes;

  - monitors the application of regulations protecting the rights of AIDS-affected children and educators;

  - establishes a culture of care in schools and their communities which can counsel, track and guide children affected by AIDS;

  - operates in more flexible (non-formal) ways: promoting subsidies for children in distress, adjusting school calendars and timetables for AIDS-affected children, establishing single-sex schools and boarding hostels, providing more 'second chance' basic education for never-schooled children, or for those whose schooling has been random;

– avoids creating a double-standard system, with special education for 'poorer' children?

- What support needs to be provided to schools-as-CBOs in the forefront of the fight against AIDS?

- What will happen to the AIDS orphans? Who will care for them and how will they be educated? Are school hostels the answer?

It is time to set out a research agenda on impact, with priorities agreed, academic and other research partners mandated and resources allocated. This needs to be done in such a way as to link research outcomes with change. The ADEA Working Group on the Teaching Profession, led by the Commonwealth Secretariat's Education Department, might provide a focus for elaborating such an agenda.

3. Responding to the Pandemic's Impact on Education
A number of things can be done at once to start coping with the impact of AIDS on the system. Some cost nothing, for they depend on committed management, planning and co-operation:

- Asserting collective dedication. Planners, their political masters, local practitioners and development agency partners can assert their collective will to understand and deal with the effect of AIDS on the education system. Common agreement is required now about factoring the influence of the pandemic into educational and cross-sectoral planning.

- Defining strategic principles. Some strategic planning principles have emerged from South Africa's experience during the 1990s:

    – Interventions must be manageable, within the capacity of the system to implement;

    – The grassroots is at work, and government policies and support mechanisms would do well to recognise that when shifting from top-down 'delivery' structures to supporting frameworks for local initiatives;

    – Peer group support is essential for all pupils, students, teachers, lecturers and other educators;

    – Collectivity, co-operation, collaboration, co-ordination and consultation, based on trust, are needed to sustain a culture of care in schools.

Such principles need to be elaborated to provide a basis for planning.

- Adapting education. It may be possible to slow down the pandemic and reduce its impact, or to circumvent its worst consequences. At the very least, it should be possible to:

    – target resources where they are most needed (for example by making provision to replace teachers lost to AIDS);

– avoid wastage (by building fewer schools where populations are decimated);

– identify at-risk student populations (female pupils, children who walk a long way to school, those in boarding hostels);

– strengthen AIDS-dedicated planning and management;

– provide a wide selection of resource materials to principals, teachers and other educators in support of peer group work;

– begin to plan for 'randomised' education and training for learners affected by AIDS.

The 1997 review of South Africa's AIDS strategy suggested that 'ensuring good STD care is simpler than organising peer education or doing outreach with marginalised groups'. It is tempting to believe that, despite the complexity of the problems now being faced, it should be possible to identify a core of actions which will save lives and protect education quality. One eminent educator has recommended concentrating not just on the 20 per cent who are affected by AIDS, but particularly on the 80 per cent or so who are still well and strong. These two concepts may provide pointers towards positive, manageable action which will make a difference.

In southern Africa, governments and their partners have tried for 20 years to stop, or at least slow and contain, the AIDS pandemic. They have failed to the extent that everyone in the region must now learn to live with AIDS. This includes children, their schools and communities, the teaching service and the education system itself. Educators can start by being aware, analysing available information, planning pragmatically, and applying tough management techniques appropriate to a crisis which is perhaps the worst yet faced by humanity.

Notes

1. Coombe, Carol (1999). *Ten-Year Plan for Educator Development and Support in Namibia.* Windhoek, Ministry of Education; HIV/AIDS and the Education Sector Strategic Plan (Mozambique); Education Sector Planning – Learning to Live with AIDS. Maputo, MINED/Irish Aid.

2. Coombe, Carol (2000). *Managing the Impact of HIV/AIDS on the Education Sector.* UNECA.

3. Kingdom of Swaziland, Ministry of Education (1999). *Impact Assessment of HIV/AIDS on the Education Sector.* JTK Associates.

4. Personal communication to author.

5. Personal communication from Dr Ko Chih Tung, Co-ordinator, ADEA Working Group on Statistics, UNESCO Regional Office/NESIS, Harare.

Bibliography

Association for the Development of Education in Africa (ADEA) (2000). Identifying Effective Responses to HIV/AIDS; Guidelines (for country case studies); Overview of the Relationships Between HIV/AIDS and Education. Letter to Ministers of Education in Africa. Paris: ADEA/IIEP.

Badcock-Walters, P and Whiteside, A (1999). *HIV/AIDS and Development in the Education Sector*. DFID Briefing Paper. Pretoria: DFID.

Barnett, T and Whiteside, A. (n.d.). *Guidelines for Preparation and Execution of Studies of the Social and Economic Impact of HIV/AIDS*. University of Natal Durban/HEARD.

Cohen, D (1999). *Responding to the Socio-Economic Impact of the HIV Epidemic in sub-Saharan Africa: Why a Systems Approach is Needed*. New York: UNDP. www.undp.org/hiv

Cohen, D (1999). 'The HIV Epidemic and the Education Sector in sub-Saharan Africa.' HIV and Development Programme Issues Paper No 32. New York: UNDP. www.undp.org/hiv

Coombe, Carol (1999). 'HIV/AIDS and the Education Sector Strategic Plan (Mozambique): Education Sector Planning – Learning to Live with AIDS'. Paper prepared for the Education Sector Strategic Plan First Annual Review Meeting, Maputo, May 1999. Maputo: MINED/Irish Aid.

Gachuhi, D (1999). 'The Impact of HIV/AIDS on Education Systems in the Eastern and Southern Africa Region, and the Response of Education Systems to HIV/AIDS: Life Skills Programmes'. Paper prepared for the sub-Saharan Africa Conference on EFA 2000, Johannesburg, December 1999. Nairobi: UNICEF Eastern and Southern Africa Regional Office.

Health Economics and HIV/AIDS Research Division, University of Natal (n.d.). *HIV/AIDS and Education: A Human Capital Issue*. Durban: University of Natal Durban/HEARD.

Kelly, M J (2000). Universities and HIV/AIDS. Terms of reference for proposed ADEA investigation in selected universities in Africa. Paris: ADEA Working Group on Higher Education.

Kelly, M J (2000). 'The Encounter between HIV/AIDS and Education', Harare, UNESCO. A synthesis of presentations to the Lusaka ICASA and the Johannesburg EFA 2000 Conferences for release at the Dakar EFA Forum.

Kelly, M J (2000). 'HIV/AIDS and Basic Education'. Paper prepared for EFA Dakar meeting, April 2000.

Kelly, M J (1999). 'What HIV/AIDS Can Do to Education, and What Education Can Do to HIV/AIDS'. Paper presented to the All sub-Saharan Africa Conference on Education for All – 2000, Johannesburg, Lusaka: University of Zambia, December 1999.

To the Edge: AIDS Review 2000. University of Pretoria Centre for the Study of AIDS, Marais, HIV/AIDS, 2000.

National Strategic Plan to Combat STD/HIV/AIDS, 2000–2002. Maputo: Ministry of Health, Mozambique, 1999.

Ten-Year Plan for Educator Development and Support in Namibia. Namibia, Ministry of Basic

Education and Culture. Windhoek: MBEC, June 1999.

HIV/AIDS in Zimbabwe: Background, Projections, Impact, Interventions. Harare: NACP, Ministry of Health and Child Welfare, Zimbabwe, 1998.

Shaeffer, S (1994). *The Impact of HIV/AIDS on Education: A Review of Literature and Experience.* Section for Preventive Education. Paris: UNESCO.

Smart, R (1999). *Children Living with HIV/AIDS in South Africa: A Rapid Appraisal.* Pretoria: Department of Health and Save the Children, UK.

The HIV/AIDS Emergency: Guidelines for Educators. Department of Education, South Africa, Pretoria, 2000.

HIV/AIDS Impact Assessment in the Education Sector in South Africa. Terms of reference for an impact assessment, prepared by the Information Systems Directorate, Department of Education, South Africa, Pretoria, 1999.

National Policy on HIV/AIDS for Learners and Educators in Public Schools, and Students and Educators in Further Education and Training Institutions of the Department of Education. In *Government Gazette,* Department of Education, Pretoria, South Africa, 10 August 1999.

Impact Assessment of HIV/AIDS on the Education Sector. Report to the Ministry of Education (Kingdom of Swaziland) by JTK Associates, Mbabane, 1999.

Whiteside, A (1999). *The Economic Impact of AIDS in Africa.* Durban. University of Natal Durban/HEARD.

Whiteside, A, ed. (1998). *Implications of AIDS for Demography and Policy in Southern Africa.* Health Economics and HIV/AIDS Research Division, University of Natal, Durban.

The Impact of HIV/AIDS on Higher Education: The Response of the Universities

Dorothy Garland

The Naked Truth

The following words of the then Deputy President of South Africa, Thabo Mbeki, in October 1998, reflect a reality that is far from unique:

For too long we have closed our eyes as a nation, hoping the truth was not so real. For many years we have allowed the human immuno-deficiency virus to spread. At times we did not know that we were burying people who had died from AIDS. At other times we knew, but chose to remain silent. We face the danger that half of our youth will not reach adulthood. Their education will be wasted, the economy will shrink. There will be a large number of sick people whom the healthy will not be able to maintain. Our dreams as a people will be shattered.

The spread of HIV/AIDS in many countries of the Commonwealth has been nurtured by fear, ignorance and silence; and thus, for far too long, nations have failed to address – or even to recognise – the impact of the pandemic on their youth, education systems, employment, economic health and national development.

The Challenge

The universities of the Commonwealth have an ethical and intellectual responsibility to set an example by openly debating these issues and finding creative responses to the threat that is posed by HIV/AIDS. It could furthermore be argued that the universities are an essential vehicle for the provision of a united and effective response to the HIV/AIDS pandemic because they have the capacity to:

- introduce strategies to contain the spread of the disease in the higher education sector and thereby ensure that, in the long term, economies are neither weakened by a diminishing supply of educated, skilled and professionally qualified young people nor deprived of future leaders;

- set standards of good practice within society as a whole in terms of both the prevention of infection and the care and support of people living with HIV/AIDS;

- give leadership to government and to the community in the development of policies which are founded on human rights and which address the whole range of political, social, economic, legal and management implications of HIV/AIDS.

But do the universities recognise this challenge? Are they even aware of the threat that the pandemic poses to their very existence?

Regional Discrepancies

In considering these questions it has to be recognised, of course, that not all Commonwealth countries are affected to the same extent by the spread of HIV/AIDS, and the statistics reveal a disturbing differential between the wealthy, industrialised countries and those that are economically disadvantaged. The following key data bear reiterating:

- It is estimated that, since the beginning of the AIDS epidemic, some 50 million individuals worldwide have been infected with HIV, of whom 33 million are still alive while 16 million have already died.

- The peoples of the Commonwealth constitute only 29.5 per cent of the world's population, yet the incidence of HIV/AIDS in Commonwealth countries accounts for 60.5 per cent of the global total.[1]

- By the end of 1997 nearly 14.5 million people in Commonwealth sub-Saharan Africa and 4.25 million in the Commonwealth countries of south and southeast Asia were estimated either to be HIV-positive or to have AIDS, whereas the combined total for Australia, Canada, New Zealand and the UK was only 81,500.[2]

- In 1998, a third of the women attending antenatal clinics in KwaZulu-Natal, South Africa, were HIV-positive.

- A 1999 survey of one tertiary institution in South Africa suggested that 25 per cent of the student body was infected with the virus.

The Impact[3]

It is clear that, within the foreseeable future, the AIDS epidemic will begin seriously to affect the enrolments, performance, staffing levels, finances and mission of large numbers of Commonwealth universities.

Enrolments

As the epidemic begins to take its toll of young people who would otherwise be eligible to enter the higher education sector, the pattern of enrolments (and of income derived therefrom) will begin to reflect the loss of this tranche of students.

Performance

Fear, anxiety, stigmatisation and increasing sickness all have the capacity to impair the performance of affected students and staff members.

Staffing Levels

As, inevitably, members of staff begin to die or become too debilitated to work, universities will be affected in particular by: 1) the need in the short term either to recruit replacement administrative and teaching staff or to redesign curricula to accommodate the staff shortages; and 2) the long-term implications of losing junior lecturing staff, from among whom the future intellectual leadership of a university is customarily nurtured and developed.

Finances

There will be cost implications related to:

• additional staff recruitment, training and development;

• the care and counselling of sick and dying staff and students;

• general health care, benefit, insurance and pension schemes;

• staff and student loan schemes (in the event that incapacity or death should occur before a loan is repaid);

• the availability of student bursaries;

• the drain on funds that might otherwise be available for expansion and development.

Mission

However their individual mission statements may be worded, universities share, on the whole, a common commitment to:

• academic excellence in teaching and research (whether pure or applied);

• the service of the societies in which they operate (through the creation and sharing of knowledge, through research and development work, and by providing tomorrow's leaders in commerce and industry, the health services, politics and government).

Both these objectives are likely to be impaired by the impact of HIV/AIDS on the staff and student body.

The Response

The Association of Commonwealth Universities (ACU) is committed to raising awareness of the implications of HIV/AIDS within the higher education sector. Professor Brenda Gourley, Vice-Chancellor of the University of Natal and former Chair of the Association's Council, first alerted the ACU to the immensity of the problem within KwaZulu-Natal; but her initial intervention stimulated the development of what has become a broad-based programme of activities from which, it is hoped, the whole of the Commonwealth university sector stands to benefit.

One such activity was a two-day seminar, held in South Africa in November 1999, at which a pan-Commonwealth group comprising experts in the field, key university staff and representatives of relevant government ministries met to consider the social, demographic and development impact of HIV/AIDS and to recommend how the universities might respond to it. Out of that meeting emerged what were held to be the core elements that should inform any university's thinking about its response and these are summarised below.

Commitment and Involvement at all Levels

If the potentially devastating impact of HIV/AIDS is to be averted, it is essential that the executive head (vice-chancellor, president, rector or principal) is fully aware of all its implications; that he/she gives leadership in encouraging the staff and student body to acknowledge and share ownership of the problems; and that all work together in finding practical and creative solutions.

Mainstreaming HIV/AIDS

As HIV/AIDS impinges on the whole fabric of society and on every aspect of institutions such as universities, it should be mainstreamed, or integrated, as an issue that demands a response at every level of a university's operations – whether related to strategic planning, teaching and research, the provision of services or the mobilisation of human and financial resources.

HIV/AIDS Policy

It can be a useful strategy to develop a policy (or to amend existing policies) specifically to embrace and address the wide range of HIV/AIDS-related issues; and, in that process, to include as many representatives of the university community as possible. (One of the outcomes of the 1999 seminar was a draft policy which ACU will be offering to its 486 member universities, and other interested parties, as a framework for consideration.)

Provision of HIV/AIDS Information, Education and Training[4]

The mainstreaming of HIV/AIDS education into the core curricula, for instance, would give all students the opportunity to:

- benefit from intellectual debate about the medical, social, demographic and economic issues relating to HIV/AIDS;

- acquire an informed understanding of how HIV and AIDS might affect their own future and professional careers;

- determine the value of modifying their behaviour in order to reduce the risk of receiving or spreading infection;

- learn about the implications of HIV/AIDS in the workplace and enter the workforce reasonably equipped to manage HIV/AIDS programmes, to deal (legally and sensitively) with colleagues and staff who are infected, and to monitor and sustain relevant workplace initiatives;

- develop an understanding of different social groups and attitudes, and a caring, tolerant and non-discriminatory approach to people living with HIV/AIDS;

- understand the potential impact of HIV/AIDS on the economic and social development of their country and region.

The difficulty, of course, lies in persuading less than enthusiastic staff of the value of incorporating what may be perceived as 'inessentials' into already overloaded courses.

Research

The relevance and value of encouraging and supporting HIV/AIDS research initiatives not only in the medical and biomedical but also social and behavioural sciences – and of disseminating the results – cannot be over-emphasised.

Care and Counselling

The provision of health care and counselling for affected staff and students carries huge cost implications. However, it is an intrinsic element of any university's objective to treat those living with HIV/AIDS in a just, humane and life-affirming way and to help them perform in their work and studies to their maximum potential.

Human Rights

Universities have a crucial leadership role to play in openly acknowledging that staff and students living with HIV/AIDS share the same rights and responsibilities as all others. This includes their right to choose not to disclose their status, to confidentiality in the handling of test results and to respect for their state of health and sexual preference.

Gender Perspective

Women are particularly susceptible to HIV/AIDS for a variety of reasons, some of which are biological while others are sociological. Examples of the latter include a false perception of their social position and hence of their right to resist coercive sex; sexual abuse and violence; and the belief in some cultures that a man infected with HIV will be cured by having sexual intercourse with a virgin. Although many countries and universities pay lip-service to gender equity, the HIV/AIDS pandemic demands real commitment to the introduction of sustainable programmes to address such inequities as exist, and to ensure that the whole university community is sensitised to the rights of women and recognises those instances in which they might be vulnerable.

Human Resource Planning and Policies

An essential element of the response to the pandemic will be a review, and possible revision, of:

- recruitment policies and personnel planning to take account of the projected numbers of sick and dying staff;

- health care, insurance and pension benefits to accommodate increasing numbers of incapacitated staff and students;

- bursaries and loan schemes to staff and students (bearing in mind the possibility of incapacity or death occurring before a loan is repaid).

Complacency

Danger lurks around many corners in the guise of complacency. In those countries where the epidemic is spreading rapidly and universities have perhaps already spent months developing an appropriate policy, there lies the danger of failing to act on that policy (as has been seen to be the case with equal opportunities policies). In other countries, where the spread of HIV infection appears to have been contained, and where life-prolonging drugs are affordable, there lies the danger of a false sense of security leading to carelessness in personal behaviour and a diminution of political incentive.

The Challenge Revisited

HIV/AIDS is no respecter of race, gender or economic status; everyone is to a greater or lesser extent vulnerable to infection. The peoples of the Commonwealth thus share on the one hand a common threat and, on the other, a common bond of responsibility for each other's welfare. The universities of the Commonwealth are in a uniquely privileged position in that, through collaboration in research and the sharing of strategies, information and experience of best practice, they have the potential to be a powerful influence for good not only within the higher education sector but also within the community at large, regionally, nationally and internationally.

Notes

1. Joint United Nations Programme on AIDS (UNAIDS) and the World Health Organization (WHO), Report on the global HIV/AIDS epidemic, June 1998. Geneva... UNAIDS/ WHO.

2. Ibid.

3. For this section I have drawn on the text of the draft HIV/AIDS Policy paper prepared by ACU in conjunction with the University of Pretoria and Abt Associates South Africa.

4. See note 3.

HIV/AIDS and Health Manifestations

Cutaneous Manifestations of HIV Infection in India

Prakash C Bora

Acquired immunodeficiency syndrome (AIDS) was recognised when Kaposi's sarcoma and pneumocystis carine were noted in young healthy homosexual men in the United States.[1] Recent reports have shown that a variety of skin diseases are commonly associated with HIV infection.[2] It is suggested that the spectrum of cutaneous manifestations occurring in AIDS cases reflect local geographic or socio-economic conditions and variations in their risk factors.[3] In India the prevalence of AIDS and sero-reactivity to HIV has been increasing steadily each year and by October 1999 89,840 HIV sero-reactive cases and 9,504 AIDS cases had been reported to the National AIDS Control Organisation, Ministry of Health, New Delhi.[4] Very few reports of cutaneous lesions in patients with AIDS are documented in the Indian literature.

It has been noted that certain skin disorders which are seen in the general population occur with increasing frequency among HIV seropositive individuals and their manifestations may be florid. Mucocutaneous changes can give valuable information to clinicians regarding systemic disorders and the immunological status of the person affected with HIV/AIDS.

Progressive decline in number and functional capacity of CD4 cells is the basic defect in the pathogenesis of HIV disease. This in turn gives rise to decreased cytotoxic responses and this is responsible for various manifestations. This altered immunity and changing pattern of infective pathogens associated with the disease progression is responsible for atypical, extensive and more severe manifestations of common skin conditions. There seems to be a correlation between degree of immunosuppression and clinical outcome of skin diseases.

HIV disease is a chronic disease with a span of 10 to 15 years. As the immunity gradually declines over a period of time, a variety of fungal, parasitic, bacterial and viral infections of skin and mucosa occur with increasing frequency.[5] Some manifestations are related to nutritional status and vitamin deficiencies. Many of the papular and papulosquamous manifestations, like lichen planus and psoriasis, are also seen commonly with different morphological presentations.

Some cutaneous conditions are commonly seen in HIV infection but may not be specific to HIV infection, for example xerosis, tinea, folliculitis and psoriasis. Some are highly suggestive of HIV, for example oral candidiasis. Some of these manifestations, alone or particularly in combination with other HIV related signs and symptoms, are fairly specific for HIV infection, while some are unique to HIV infection, for example hairy leukoplakia of the tongue or disseminated Kaposi's sarcoma.

Classification

Classification of various cutaneous manifestations can be done in many ways, for example aetiological, regional or according to the stage of the disease. I would like to put forward a classification based on manifestations in different stages as well as aetiological factors, which would enable clinicians to appreciate their diagnostic and prognostic significance. In the late symptomatic and AIDS stage 50 per cent of patients have manifestations of more than two conditions. In a study conducted in Lusaka, one or more cutaneous lesions occurred in 98 per cent of AIDS patients as compared to 53 per cent of those with ARC.[6]

Predominant cutaneous manifestations in various stages of HIV/AIDS in India

Skin disorder		Stage*	
	Early symptomatic stage	Early symptomatic stage	AIDS
Infection			
Viral	Herpes zoster, Herpes Simplex	Herpes Zoster, Herpes Simplex, Condyloma acuminata	Extra genital Molluscum contagiosum, Oral Hairy Leukoplakia, Herpetic oral ulcers, CMV infection
Bacterial	Recurrent pyoderma	Foliculitis, atypical pyoderma	Atypical mycobacteriosis
Fungal	Tinea versicolor, Tinea corporis	Dermatophytosis, Onychomycosis, Tinea corporis	Oral candidiasis, Disseminated candidiasis, Cryptococcal infection, Histoplasmosis
Protozoal			Toxoplasmosis, Amoebiasis
Parasitic	Scabies	Scabies	Norwegian scabies
Papulo squamous	Acne, Lichen planus, Pruritic papular eruption	Psoriasis, Seborrheic dermatitis, Pruritic papular eruption, Reiter's disease	Recalcitrant seborrheic dermatitis, Pruritic papular eruption, prurigo nodularis
Vascular		Thrombocytopenic purpura	Deep vein thrombosis
Neoplasm		Squamous cell carcinoma	Squamous cell carcinoma, Basal cell carcinoma, Kaposi's sarcoma, Non Hodgkin lymphoma

Skin disorder		Stage*	
	Early symptomatic stage	Early symptomatic stage	AIDS
Infection			
Nutritional Deficiencies		Asteatosis, Angular chelitis, Pellagra	Hyperpigmentation, Pellagra, Icthiosis, Xerosis
Hair and nail changes		Dry hair, hair loss, lustreless nails	Lustreless hair, brittle nails, yellow nails
Oral manifestations		Apthosis, gingivitis, periodontal disease	Oral hairy leukoplakia, oral candidiasis
Miscellaneous	Drug reaction	Pruritus, fixed drug eruption, erythema multiforme, Stevens Johnson's syndrome	Drug eruption, erythema multiforme, Stevens Johnson's syndrome

*Some overlapping can occur in different stages.

The Indian Scenario

It has been well documented that diseases most commonly encountered in patients with AIDS are caused by agents/pathogens that are endemic to specific regions.[7,9] The pattern of skin lesions in Indian patients with HIV infection may be different from that in the West.[3] It is important to note the significant epidemiologic differences regarding cutaneous manifestations in AIDS cases in India, the Western countries and Africa.

Limited data are available on the prevalence of skin diseases in patients with HIV infection in India. Various workers have reported different cutaneous manifestations in Indian HIV-positive patients.[3,8,11–19, 21–23]

A clinical study from southern India noted that inflammatory skin lesions occur among 38 per cent (excluding oral candidiasis).[3] The African study showed infectious skin lesions in the range of 28–60 per cent.[5]

Thirty-two HIV-positive patients were screened for cutaneous and oral lesions and matched controls of the same age and sex from an HIV-negative group were compared. In this study from a rural medical college prevalence of oral candidiasis, icthiosis, alopecia and scabies was reported to be significantly higher.[11]

Another study of 15 cases of papular eruption in HIV patients was complemented with skin biopsies. Histopathological examination revealed eosinophillic infiltration. Pruritic papular eruption can be the most common and early manifestation.[12]

Herpes Zoster is frequently reported among HIV seropositive patients presenting as multidermatomal, recurrent, necrotic, bullous or haemorrhageic lesions and is associated with delayed healing.[16]

Four cases of disseminated infection caused by penicilium marnefei in HIV-infected patients are documented from the Indian state of Manipur.[19]

Histopathological analysis of cutaneous lesions in HIV/AIDS was carried out by Lanjewar and colleagues in Mumbai (Bombay). A total of 195 skin biopsies were examined: 180 showed significant microscopic findings; 104 (53 per cent) cases were comprised of skin infections; 66 (34 per cent) of miscellaneous skin conditions; and 12(6 per cent) of cutaneous neoplasms. Among skin infections molluscum contagiosum and cutaneous tuberculosis were seen in more numbers. Squamous cell carcinoma was diagnosed in 9 out of 12 cases of cutaneous malignancies. Psoriasis was observed in 21 out of 66 cases of miscellaneous skin conditions.[20] Although most African and Western studies show a high incidence of Kaposi's sarcoma associated with HIV infection, there are only three reports of Kaposi's sarcoma published in the Indian literature.[15]

Of 1,434 HIV seropositive patients seen in my practice between 1994 and 1999, 410 (28.6 per cent) presented with cutaneous manifestations. Of those 410 patients, 261 had Herpes Zoster, 10 with extra genital molluscum; 73 had oral candidiasis; 8 had erosive herpes simplex; 12 had oral hairy leukoplakia; and 4 had Norwegian scabies. Hair and nail changes were seen in 25 per cent of patients. Lichen planus, psoriasis, seborheic dermatitis, pruritic papular eruption and Reiters disease were other papulosquamous skin conditions encountered in these patients.[17]

In a study reported from Chennai dental college, the oral lesions reported are oral candidiasis (56 per cent), gingivitis (50 per cent), periodontitis (9.5 per cent), oral ulcers (3 per cent), oral hairy leukoplakia (1 per cent), in a series of 200 patients.[21]

Clinical Features and Treatment

Although cutaneous infections form a major portion of reported skin conditions, inflammatory dermatoses or papulo squamous conditions and cutaneous neoplasms are also significantly increased in HIV disease.

Infections
Viral Infections
Herpes Simplex
Herpes simplex usually presents as severe and recurrent vesicular eruption. Patients with HIV disease often have persistent manifestation of HSV and require higher

doses of acyclovir for an extended length of time than is recommended for immuno-competent hosts.

Herpes Zoster

Unilateral painful eruption of grouped vesicles along one or more dermatomes is characteristic. Herpes zoster seen in young individuals is a cutaneous marker of HIV infection and therefore questions about high-risk behaviour should be asked of those individuals and screening should be done for HIV infection. In studies conducted at ARCON in Sir J. J. Hospital in Mumbai (Bombay), prepondarance of thoracic, opthalmic, and lumbosacral dermatomes was seen in decreasing order of frequency. Multidermatomal herpes with necrotic lesions is seen at the stage of AIDS.[22]

Ophthalmic zoster is seen more frequently in HIV patients and severe forms can cause corneal ulceration and consequent blindness. It is therefore important to start acyclovir in higher dosage along with corticosteroids very early to prevent scarring and disfigurement. VZ infections also require higher doses of acyclovir.

Warts

Human Papilloma virus infection or warts are common and are best treated by locally destructive measures like cryotherapy, topical agents like tretinoin .05 per cent cream or topical fluorouracil cream once or twice daily.

Condyloma Acuminata

Condyloma acuminata presents as florid warty growths and usually responds to the application of podohyllum resin 25 per cent in benzoin applied weekly till the lesions resolve. Continuous application may be required. One needs to rule out development of squamous cell carcinoma in recalcitrant lesions of condyloma acuminata.

Molluscum Contagiosum

Molluscum contagiosum is characterised by central umbilication of wart-like papular eruptions. Extensive extra-genital molluscum contagiosum in adult patients should give rise to suspicion of HIV infection. The lesions are extensive, multiple and occur at unusual sites, for example eyelids.

Molluscum contagiosum is a severe problem in patients with HIV infection especially when the CD4 T cell counts fall below 250/mm. Liquid nitrogen cryosurgery or topical tretinoin cream or 5 per cent rifampicin paste is beneficial.

Bacterial Infections

Most bacterial infections are caused by Staphylococcus. They respond to a prolonged course of appropriate antibiotics. Cutaneous atypical mycobacterial infections are rarely encountered and they respond to minocyline 100mg or clarithromycin 500mg orally twice daily.

Fungal Infections

Candidiasis

Candidiasis is one of the most common opportunistic infections seen in HIV disease. Profuse curd-like lesions on the tongue, palate, buccal mucosa are common presentation in the stage of AIDS. The palate, oesophagus and pharynx are commonly involved and may cause dysphagia or pain on swallowing. It usually responds well to systemic and topical antifungal therapy with fluconazole 200mg daily for 14 days.

Dermatophytosis

Tinea versicolor may be more severe and extensive than usually observed. Extensive dematophytosis, onychomycosis would require systemic oral anti-fungal agents like iatroconazole or fluconazloe.

Cryptococcal Infection

Cryptococcal infection may present occasionally with molluscum like or herpetiform lesions.[23,24] Diagnosis can be confirmed by histopathological examination and India ink preparation. Thrombo-phlebitis or deep vein thrombosis is sometimes observed secondary to deep mycoses.

Parasitic Infections

Scabies

Scabies is commonly observed with generalised pruritus, and papules and burrows in interdigital areas and axillary folds, inner thighs and lower abdomen. Norwegian scabies is seen more commonly in AIDS with intense pruritis, and crusted lesions on palms and on the trunk.

Non-infectious Disorders

Drug Reactions

Drug reactions, more commonly associated with generalised pruritus, fixed drug eruptions, erythema multiforme and Stevens-Johnsons's (S-J) Syndrome, are seen with more frequency in HIV-positive individuals. Thiacetazone is contra-indicated in HIV patients due to the likelihood of developing life-threatening S-J Syndrome. Drug reactions are commonly seen with sulfa, penicillin and anti-tubercular medicines.

Pruritic Papular Eruption

Pruritic papular eruption presents as intensely pruritic, papular, or necrotic lesions. Papules, scratch lesions, and hyperpigmented macules are symmetrically distributed over the body, more frequently on extremities. Histological features are non-specific and include perivascular infiltration with mononuclear cells and eosinophils. In populations with high infection rates, the diagnostic accuracy of the papular eruption is very high.

Prurigo Nodularis

Prurigo nodularis may develop in patients with HIV infection presenting as multiple pruritic nodules on extremities. Routine anti-pruritic measures and doxepin ointment locally or topical steroids are useful.

Seborrhoeic Dermatitis

Seborrhoeic dermatitis has been reported by several authors to occur with greater frequency and severity in patients with HIV infection.[25] The appearance may vary from mild to more extensive reddening and scaling of the face. Demodex folliculorum may be present in greater number than normal in some cases. It may or may not respond to topical steroids but may require oral ketoconazole or iatroconazole in some cases.

Psoriasis

It presents as extensive silvery scaly lesions on the scalp and extremities. Psoriasis may be difficult to control in HIV patients and isotretinoin in doses of 40 mg once or twice daily coupled with UV-B phototherapy may be useful.

Reiter's Disease

Reiter's disease may present as keratotic lesions on palm and soles, and psoriasiform lesions on the trunk and involvement of conjuctival and genital mucosa. Large doses of oral steroids and antibiotics are required.

Xerosis and Icthiosis

Xerosis and icthiosis are commonly seen in AIDS patients. Xerosis is more generalised while icthiosis occurs more on lower extremities. Seborrheic dermatitis may also be seen along with xerosis, and icthiosis. These patients usually have weight loss and cachexia. Nutritional deficiencies may be the contributing factors in those conditions.

Nails

Nails show loss of lustre and brittleness. Yellow nail changes are very characteristic of HIV infection showing yellowish discolouration of the distal part of nails.

Hair

Hair is usually dry and lustreless in the late stages of the HIV disease. There may be extensive hair loss secondary to nutritional deficiencies or seborrheic dermatitis.

Pigmentation

Hyperpigmentation of face and extremities is commonly seen in terminally ill AIDS patients. Pellagrinous dematitis may be encountered in a few of these patients.

Cutaneous Neoplasms

Squamous cell carcinomas are more common than basal cell carcinoma and Kaposi's sarcoma as reported in western literature. HIV-associated Kaposi's Sarcoma is very rare in Indian subjects. At present, only three cases have been reported.[13–15] Sometimes occurrence of non-Hodgkin's cutaneous lymphoma is seen in association with HIV infection.

Oral Manifestations

The oral manifestations include oral candidiasis, herpes virus ulcerations, hairy leukoplakia, rapidly progressive periodontal disease, gingivitis, or recurrent apthous type ulcers and xerostomia.

Oral lesions in HIV Infection

Oral hairy leukoplakia
Candidiasis
Herpes Simplex
Apthous type ulcers
Xerostomia
Gingivitis
Periodontal disease
Warts

Apthous stomatitis

Extensive apthosis presents as recurrent, painful ulcers on the upper lip and tip of tongue or sides of tongue. They are recalcitrant and respond to higher dosage of locally-acting steroids. One should also rule out herpetic ulcers.

Oral Hairy Leukoplakia

Oral hairy leukoplakia presents as slightly raised, poorly demarcated lesions with corrugated surface on the lateral borders of the tongue. Epstein Barr virus is supposed to be the aetiological factor and often does not require treatment. Unlike plaques of oral candidiasis, lesions of hairy leukoplakia cannot be scraped off. It can be treated with local application of topical podophyllum 20 per cent in alcohol used once or twice daily.

Periodontal Disease

Periodontal disease is characterised by gingival recession with marked gingival inflammation and rapid alveolar bone loss.

Acute Necrotising Gingivitis

Acute necrotising gingivitis presents as painful, erythematous, swollen gingivia and spontaneous gingival bleeding, and necrosis of interdental papilla with greyish necrotic slough.

Conclusion

Certain cutaneous manifestations serve as markers of HIV/AIDS while others give information about the possible stage of disease. Thus, skin manifestations have significant diagnostic and prognostic value. It is very important to know about these cutaneous and oral manifestations which may enable the clinician to suspect, screen, diagnose and assess the state of the patient.

References

1. Hymes, K B, Cheung, T, Greene, J B et al. (1981). 'Kaposi's Sarcoma in Homosexual Men: A Report of Eight Cases', *Lancet* 2: 598–603.

2. Smith, K J, Skelton, H G, Yeager, J et al. (1994). 'Cutaneous findings in HIVpositive patients. A 42 month prospective study', *Journal of the American Academy of Dermatology* 31: 746–54.

3. Rajgopalan, B, Jacob, M and Geirge, S (1996). 'Skin lesions in HIV positive and HIV negative patients in South India', *International Journal of Dermatology* 35: 489–92.

4. National AIDS Control Program: India – country scenario. An update surveillance of HIV infection in India, 1986 to October1999. New Delhi: National AIDS Control Organisation in India, Ministry of Health and family welfare, Government of India. 1999.

5. Ansary, M A, Hira, S K, Bayley, A C, Chintu, C and Nyaywa, C L. Cutaneous Manifestation AIDS in the Tropic Colour Atlas, p. 28.

6. Hira, S K, Wadhawan, D, Kamanga, J et al. (1988). 'Cutaneous manifestation of human deficiency virus in Lusaka, Zambia', *Journal of the American Academy of Dermatology* 19: 451–7.

7. Lanjewar, D N, Anand, B S, Genta, R et al. (1996). 'Major differences in the spectrum of gastrointestinal infections associated with AIDS in versus the West. An autopsy study', *Clin Infec Dis* 23: 482–5.

8. Singh, A, Thappa, D M and Hamide, A (1999). 'The spectrum of mucocutaneous manifestations during the evolutionary phases of HIV disease: an emerging scenario', *Journal of Dermatology* 26: (5) 294–304.

9. Selik, R M, Starcher, E T and Curran, J W (1987). 'Opportunistic diseases reported in AIDS patients: Frequencies, associations and trends', *AIDS* 1: 175–82.

10. Goodman, D S, Tepitz, E D et al. (1987). 'Prevalence of cutaneous disease in patients with AIDS or AIDS related complex', *Journal of the American Academy of Dermatology* 17: 210–20.

11. Rajgopal, S, Chidambaram, P, Ramprasad, T and Ponnusamy, Manoharan G (2000). *Study of cutaneous manifestations of AIDS from January 1999 to October 1999 in rural medical college.* AIDS INDIA. Book abstract, p. 19.

12. Murugusundaram, S, Kumarsamy, N, Solomon, S and Yesudian, P (2000). *Pruritic papular eruption in persons with HIV.* AIDS INDIA. Book abstract, p. 23.

13. Kumarswamy, N, Solomon, S, Yesudian, P and Surgumar, P (1996). 'First report of Kaposi's sarcoma in an AIDS patient from Madras India', *Indian Journal of Dermatology* 41: 23–25.

14. Ganesh, R, Williams, J, Uma, A et al. (1991). 'AIDS and Kaposi's Sarcoma in a French passive homosexual', *Indian J Sex Transim Dis* 1236–37.

15. Shroff, H J, Dashatwar, D R, Deshpande, R P and Waigmann, H R (1993). 'AIDS associated Kaposi's sarcoma in an Indian female', *JAPI* 41 (4) 242–2.

16. Saple, D G et al. *Dermavision beyond 2000*. Indian National Conference. Book abstract, p. 19.

17. Bora, P. Cutaneous manifestations in 1434 cases of HIV-AIDS from Jan 1994 to Dec1999. Unpublished.

18. Khopkar, U, Raj, S, Sukhankar, A, Kulkarni, M G and Wadhwa, S L (1992). 'Clinical profile of HIV infection', *Ind J Dermatolo Venerol Leprol*, 58: 155–8.

19. Ngh, P N, Ranjana, K, Singh, Y I et al. (1999). 'Indigenous disseminated Penicillum Marnefei infection in the state of Manipur, India. Report of four autochthonus cases', *J Clin Microbiol* 37(8): 2699–702.

20. Newar, D N, Bhosale, A, Iyer, A et al. *Cutaneous lesions in HIV-AIDS*. National Conference. IAPM. Book abstract.

21. Nanathan, K, Uma, D et al. (2000). *Oral and maxillofacial lesions among 200 patients with HIV-AIDS in Chennai, India*. AIDS India. Book abstract, p. 32.

22. CON Training manual, p. 8.

23. Walwshwarkar, S N, Medhekar, S V, Saple, D G and Maniar, J K. *Dermatological presentations of Histoplasmosis, Cryptococosis and Aspergillosis in HIV/AIDS, Dermavision beyond 2000*. Book abstract, (P122], p. 162.

24. Anjewar, N, Shroff, H J, Kohli, M A and Hira, S K (1998). 'Cutaneous cryptococcosis and mollusscum contagiosum occuring in the same lesion in a patient with AIDS', *Ind J Dermatol Venerol Leprol* 64: 25–8.

The Evolving HIV/AIDS Pandemic and its Impact on Oral Health

Prince Akpabio, Sudeshni Naidoo and Usuf Chikte

The HIV pandemic continues to be a serious and catastrophic public health problem. The consequences include a rise in HIV-related morbidity with a concomitant increase in the demand for health care. Over 30 million adults and children live with HIV/AIDS.

A wide range of opportunistic infections, many of which manifest orally, are characteristic complications of HIV infections. These conditions cause pain, discomfort and eating restrictions. Oral lesions are among the first symptoms of HIV infection and HIV may herald the progression of the disease to full-blown AIDS. Early detection of HIV-related oral lesions can lead to diagnosis of HIV infection, elucidate progression of the disease, predict immune status and enable timely therapeutic intervention. The early diagnosis, treatment and management of oral HIV lesions can considerably improve the patient's well-being. The purpose of this article is to provide an overview of the evolving HIV/AIDS pandemic in the Commonwealth and to set the stage for a more detailed discussion of its impact on oral health.

Current and Future Situation of HIV/AIDS in the Commonwealth

The spread of human immunodeficiency virus (HIV) in the early 1980s has created a global pandemic with devastating consequences. The epidemic was first noted in a mainly adult, male, homosexual community in the midst of the most affluent societies in the world. Its consequences reign most terribly now in the heterosexual community, affecting men, women and children, in Commonwealth countries characterised by extensive poverty.

Most HIV-infected women and children in the Commonwealth live in the countries of sub-Saharan Africa. The annual increase of individuals infected with HIV worldwide is approaching 20 per cent. The situation in sub-Saharan Africa remains bleak. Two out of every three persons in the world with HIV/AIDS live in Africa. The likelihood of adults in Africa being infected is 10 times higher than in North America and 20 times greater than in Europe.

Southern Africa is the epicentre of the pandemic and will see a doubling of HIV-related mortality in the next few years. South Africa, with an estimated prevalence of infection ranging from 6–26 per cent, has the fastest growing epidemic in the world. The Caribbean is the second most affected region in the world after sub-Saharan Africa. India has the largest number of infected individuals (4 million) in a single country. In some Commonwealth countries, however, success in the slowing of the growth of the epidemic in some of the groups most vulnerable to its effects have been recorded, with Australia, Canada, Uganda and the UK being notable examples.

Data from several countries demonstrate a rapid rise in infection in very young women. Of every 10 women living with HIV, 8 are in Africa. In some areas of South Africa, one in three pregnant women is HIV-positive. Child-bearing women who are infected through heterosexual transmission constitute the main source of paediatric HIV infections. Evidence suggests that around 30 per cent of infants born to HIV-infected mothers in most African countries will also be infected. Vertical (mother-to-child) transmission can occur in several ways: maternal bodily fluids during labour and delivery; breast feeding; or by crossing the placenta early in gestation.

Of the 1.2 million children (under 15 years old) estimated to be living with HIV/AIDS at the end of 1998, 1 million are in Africa (83 per cent). Of the 2.5 million adult deaths from HIV/AIDS during 1998, 80 per cent (2 million) were in Africa. HIV/AIDS is now the biggest single cause of death in Africa, and has moved up to fourth place worldwide. In many countries adult life expectancy has declined, while child mortality rates have increased, demonstrating a reversal of the hard-won gains achieved in child survival and bringing about a steady increase in the number of children orphaned.

The Impact of the Epidemic on Oral Health
Importance and Relevance of Oral Lesions in HIV/AIDS

Several studies have documented the importance and relevance of oral lesions in HIV infection. Oral lesions are described as:

- the initial presenting sign of HIV infection;
- early clinical features of the disease;
- being predictive of progression of disease;
- being useful in staging and classification schemes.

In addition, oral HIV lesions are useful indicators in HIV/AIDS therapy and vaccine trials and in anti-HIV and anti-opportunistic infection therapy.

Oral lesions such as candidiasis, herpetic ulcers and Kaposi's sarcoma are among the first symptoms of HIV infection. These common oral HIV lesions are treatable with simple interventions, although if they go untreated they may lead to severe pain, discomfort or loss of masticatory function, with subsequent malnutrition, which compromises an already ill patient even further. Studies have shown that the presence of oral HIV contributes to an overall deterioration in the patient's quality of life, including lowered self-esteem and stigmatisation.

HIV-infected patients utilise health care facilities and are being treated in dental and other health care settings. Often patients are unaware of or do not divulge their HIV status. Therefore, knowledge of HIV infection has become a critically important requirement both for the patient and for all health care workers. Experience has shown that there is a need for combined education, training and understanding of HIV. Often oral lesions associated with HIV infection may be the presenting complaint, requiring expertise in oral health for diagnosis and treatment. Oral lesions can be the first sign and/or symptom of HIV infection. An increase in frequency or severity of many oral lesions in HIV-positive patients can reflect a declining immune competency, ineffectiveness of treatment or progression of the terminal phase.

Treatment of HIV patients has raised the real and emotional concerns of oral health care workers regarding their own safety and transmission risks. Ethical and legal guidelines mandate against discrimination in providing services for known or suspected HIV-positive individuals. In addition to HIV infection, there are many other transmissible infectious diseases that may pose a risk, such as tuberculosis, hepatitis and herpes.

Strategies to Reduce the Spread and Impact of Oral HIV

Oral examination is quick and inexpensive and may be appropriate, especially in screening populations at greater risk of HIV, particularly those attending genito-urinary medicine clinics. In addition, due to the location, accessibility and visibility of oral lesions, self-examination needs to be encouraged.

In areas of high HIV prevalence, diagnosis of mucosal disease may predict HIV infection in women and may be useful in antenatal screening so that appropriate drug management can be instituted to reduce vertical transmission. Many health professionals, including oral health care workers, are not familiar with oral manifestations of HIV infection. If health care workers are to screen for oral manifestations of HIV infection they will need training to identify the lesions.

Many studies have shown that oral lesions are more common in HIV-infected patients (Scully et al, 1991a; Scully et al, 1991b; Scully and Cawson; Greenspan et al, 1992). In the African region, studies have been carried out by Morgan et al (Uganda, 1998), Emodi and Okafor (Nigeria, 1998), Ticklay et al (Zimbabwe, 1997), Malkin (Burkina Faso, 1997), Leroy et al (Rwanda, 1995), Miller et al (Tanzania, 1995), Melbye et al (Zambia, 1986), Mayanja et al (Uganda, 1999), Arendorf et al (South Africa, 1998), Johnson et al (Zimbabwe, 1998), Hodgson (Zambia, 1997), Wanzala and Pindborg (Kenya, 1995) Schiodt et al (Tanzania, 1990) and Wanzala et al (Kenya, 1989). The following oral lesions have been recorded in these studies:

a) *Oral candidiasis* – very common and a very early symptom of HIV infection. A creamy white lace-like lesion in the inside of the cheek or palate. Easily removable. Requires very early detection and treatment.

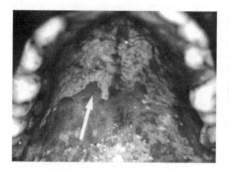

Pseudomembranous Candidiasis   *Erythematous Candidiasis*

b) *Oral herpes infection* – commonly seen in HIV-infected patients. It has a tendency to recur, usually on the lips, and requires specialist diagnosis and treatment.

c) *Oral ulceration* – lesions resemble severe persistent recurrent apthous ulcers and tend to occur in the mouth. They are often resistant to simple normal treatment and need specialist diagnosis and treatment.

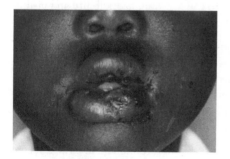
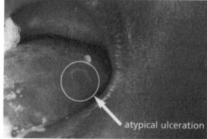

Recurrent Severe Ulceration   *Atypical Severe Ulceration*

d) *Peridontal (gum lesions)* – severe and very persistent and resistant to normal gum treatment. Needs further biopsy investigation.

e) *Hairy leukoplaka* – invariably diagnostic of HIV infection. White non-removable lesions almost invariably bilateral (i.e. on either side) of the tongue. Difficult to remove.

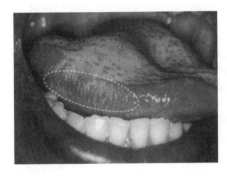
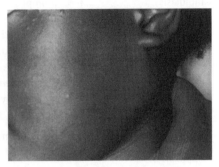

Hairy Leukoplaka   *Cervical Lymphadenopathy and Parotid enlargement*

f) *Karposi's Sarcoma.* Like hairy leukoplakia, almost invariably diagnostic of HIV infection. Occurs as isolated purple macules leading to isolated nodules, seen mainly in the hard palate. Needs specialist investigation by biopsy. May require chemotherapy under specialist care.

g) *Cervical lymphadenopathy* – enlargement of the cervical lymph nodes in HIV infection is common, although most of the literature from Africa does not report on cervical lymphadenopathy, but rather on the generalised lymphatic enlargements. Nevertheless it is something to look out for.

Benefits of dental treatment include:

- reduction of pain and sepsis;

- improvement in the function of the oral cavity (affecting eating, salivary flow, speech, aesthetics and general well-being);

- improvement of general nutritional status;

- alleviation of the debilitating effects of oral HIV mucosal lesions;

- minimising of cross-infection among patients and between patients and health care providers.

Management of Common Oral Manifestations of HIV

Oral Manifestation	Comments
Candidiasis	Treat promptly and vigorously. Due to high sugar content of some formulations, topical fluoride should be used, if frequently prescribed. Chlorhexidine gluconate (0.2 per cent) oral rinses useful – NB chlorhexidine and nystatin should *not* be used at the same time. Remove dentures when using medication. Eliminate local contributory factors like continuous denture wear, denture hygiene, xerostomia.
Herpes virus infections	Very useful if administered early. Viruses may occasionally become resistant. Treat recurrences aggressively.
Apthous ulcerations	NB Chlorhexidine should not be used at the same time with topical steroids or antifungals. If ulcers persists, despite treatment, biopsy required. Gentian violet may be useful. Successful treatment with Thalidomide has been reported – not for pregnant women.
Periodontal and gingival lesions	Oral hygiene: brushing, flossing, mouthrinses, Mobile teeth may need to be splinted or extracted. Sequestration: should be removed under antibiotic cover.
Kaposi's sarcoma	Radiation causes mucositis and xerostomia. Benzydamine hydrochloride. Systemic chemotherapy may be indicated. Good oral hygiene and plaque control to prevent secondary infection.
Xerostomia	Preventive care and dietary control are essential to avoid caries.
Caries	Preventive care, fluoride applications and dietary control are essential.

Conclusion

HIV/AIDS is a widespread problem in the Commonwealth affecting men, women and children. It is exacting a devastating toll on morbidity and mortality and has a hugely negative impact on the quality of life. It has eroded the social, political and economic health gains of the entire region; dealing with its consequences is one of the greatest challenges facing us in the new millennium.

The uniqueness of the HIV/AIDS pandemic in the under-developed countries of the Commonwealth is characterised by its heterosexual spread, its prevalence in men, women and children, the rapid rise of infection in very young women and the associated risk of vertical transmission. The severity, progression, morbidity and mortality of HIV/AIDS is fuelled by endemic poverty, malnutrition, gender inequality, and sexual and cultural practices in the region.

Oral lesions occur in symptomatic and asymptomatic HIV-infected individuals and can present as the initial sign of HIV infection or as early clinical features. In addition, they may serve as useful predictors of the progression of the disease and may be used in staging and classification schemes. Oral examinations can play a vital role in the early detection, diagnosis and management of HIV/AIDS. These examinations are simple, inexpensive and non-invasive. Many African health professionals, including dentists, are not familiar with the oro-facial signs of HIV infection. Health care workers require training to understand, diagnose, manage and research these manifestations. Effective methods of treatment, including the use of traditional medicines and palliation of oral symptoms, need to be investigated.

References available on request.

Chest Infections – An Indian Perspective

Janak Maniar

Introduction

In India, the HIV/AIDS epidemic is now more than 13 years old. Within this short period it has emerged as one of the most serious public health problems in the country. The first cases of HIV/AIDS in India were reported amongst commercial sex workers in Mumbai and Chennai and amongst injecting drug users (IDUs) in the northeastern states of India.[1] The epidemic has spread rapidly in the areas adjoining these focus points and by 1997, Maharashtra,[2] Tamil Nadu and Manipur together accounted for over three-quarters of AIDS cases and over two-thirds of HIV infections in India, with Maharashtra reporting almost half the number of cases in the country.[4]

Even though the officially reported number of cases of HIV infections and full-blown AIDS cases are only in the thousands, it is acknowledged that a wide gap exists between reported and existing cases because of the under-reporting of epidemiological data in many parts of the country.[4] It is not compulsory to report HIV-positive individuals either to the National AIDS Control Organisation (NACO) or to state health officials. One conservative estimate of the HIV-infected population in India estimated that 1.5 per cent of the one billion Indian population, or 11.5 million individuals in 1997, are already infected with HIV, which makes India the country with the largest number of HIV-infected people in the world.[5] The nationwide sentinel surveillance data collected in February–March 1998 confirmed that HIV infection is now prevalent in all parts of the country and has spread from urban to rural populations and from individuals involved with high-risk behavior to the general population.[4]

Transmission of HIV in India

About 80 per cent of infection occurs through the sexual route,13 predominantly heterosexual but also homosexual, 8 per cent through blood transfusion with infected blood, 8 per cent through injecting drug use and the remaining 4 per cent through unknown routes.[4,3] In all, over 90 per cent of the reported cases are occurring in sexually active individuals, most of whom fall within the economically productive age group of 15–45 years. One in every three cases reported is female.

In HIV disease almost every system of the body is affected, including the constitutional system.[4]

Immunology *immune complex reaction*	100%
Opthalmology *eye involvement*	30%
Constitutional symptoms *viz fever, weight loss, weakness, tiredness*	96%
Articulator system *joint and bones involvement, rheumatic infection*	20%
Respiratory system *chest infection*	90%
Oto rhino laryngology *ear, nose and throat involvement*	10%
Hematology manifestions *blood changes*	80%
Nephrology	7%
Stomatology	80%
Metabolic disorders	5%
Dermatological markers *skin diseases*	78%
Genito urinary system	2%
Gastrointestinal system	65%
Cardiovascular system	1.5 %
Central nervous system	60 %
Oncology manifestations *opportunistic cancers*	0.125%
Venereology markers *sexually transmitted infection*	40%
Peripheral vascular system	0.125 %
Psychiatric manifestions *psychological symptoms*	40%
Endocrinopathy	n.a.

Clinical Spectrum of Opportunistic Infections

The spectrum of opportunistic infections (OIs) [9,14] is almost the same throughout India with slight variations between provinces, for example Penicillium marnefei (fungal infection) has begun to appear in the northeastern provinces of India near the Golden Triangle, for example in Manipur, Nagaland and Mizoram. The commonest opportunistic infections seen are:[10,14] tuberculosis, candidiasis (oral/ oesophageal), herpes zoster, herpes simplex (reactivation), oral hairy leukoplakia, pyoderma, cryptococcosis, toxoplasmosis, cytomegalovirus retinitis, tinea, scabies, bacterial pneumonia, diarrhoea rhea, Pneumocystis carinii pneumonia (PCP), histoplamosis disseminatum and Penicilium marnefei. More than one opportunistic infection in an individual at a given time is not uncommon. Recurrence of the same OI is common in a natural history of HIV infection. Drug resistant OI over a period of time is not uncommon, which could be dangerous for life. In spite of basic counselling given to HIV-positive individuals the compliance for treatment of OI is inadequate due to various factors: financial constraint, side-effects due to treatment, carelessness or callousness, psychosocial issues, unexplained reasons, etc. There is no doubt that early recognition of OIs and their prompt treatment offer the greatest advantages to an individual, especially in resource-poor settings.

Timely initiation of antiretroviral therapy, as and when indicated, has distinct advantages for preventing and eliminating incidence of OIs. The various episodes of OIs have an adverse effect on a natural history of HIV disease; the immune system is adversely affected, the viral replication (multiplication) is stimulated resulting in significantly increased morbidity and mortality, daily wages loss, psychosocial effect, family distortion or disturbances, and the brunt of the cost of treatment including hospitalisation, if any. The limited number of studies in India have proved that the annual cost of treating OIs is much higher than that of antiretroviral therapy.

Chest Infection

The clinical spectrum of opportunistic chest infection in HIV disease in India includes: tuberculosis, bacterial pneumonia, pneumocystis carinni pneumonia (PCP), fungal infections (for example, aspergillosis, cryptocaccosis, histoplasmosis, penicillium marnfei and candida), cytomegalovirus infection.

Tuberculosis

Tuberculosis is the commonest OI, estimated to occur in 90 per cent of individuals suffering from HIV,[14] with incidence of pulmonary TB at 50 per cent, extrapulmonary TB at 50 per cent and disseminated TB at 15–20 per cent. More than one episode of TB occurs in over 60 per cent of HIV-positive people. Compliance with anti-TB treatment is < 40 per cent, which is unsatisfactory.[9] The incidence of multidrug resistant tuberculosis is on the rise. There is frequent occurrence of anti-TB drug-induced side-effects, for example, gastritis 35 per cent, hepatitis 30 per cent, and skin rashes 7 per cent. The duration of treatment with anti-tuberculosis drugs is a minimum of nine months, but it can be as long as 18 months if there is central nervous system or bone tuberculosis. Co-infection occurs sometimes with pneumonaystis carinii pneumonia, bacterial infection, candida, etc. Tuberculosis is the commonest cause of death resulting from HIV infection and it is also the commonest cause of fever of unknown origin in HIV-positive individuals. The incidence of HIV seropositivity in patients with tuberculosis varies between 10 per cent and 45 per cent.[6,12,14] Tuberculosis chest infection occurs as follows: infiltration, pleural effusion, milliary tuberculosis, consolidation, TB empyema, endobroncheal TB, perihilar pneumonia, nodular shadows, cavitatory lesion, hilar lymphadenopathy, mediastinal lymphadenopathy, pericardial effusion.

To diagnose tuberculosis of the chest, X-ray examination is not always sufficient. Sometimes a CT scan is of supplementary help; sputum examination for acid fast bacilli by Ziehl Neelson technique and direct immunofluorescence are also helpful. Culture of sputum is not done as a routine unless multidrug resistant tuberculosis is suspected. In countries like India, where tuberculosis is endemic, there is no purpose served in isolating chest TB patients or putting them in a negative pressure room. The Mantoux test or tuberculin test is invariably negative in HIV-positive individuals having manifest tuberculosis infection. In asymptomatic HIV-positive individuals having reactive MT between 5–10 mm, the use of two drug prophylaxis, rifampicin[11] and isoniazide is advocated for at least six months. Recent recommendation of chemoprophylaxis in combination of rifampician and pyrizinamide for six weeks is under study for its efficacy. Our studies have demonstrated the failure of chemoprophylaxis by rifampicin plus isonizid for six months (600 patients) and TB chemoprophylaxis is no longer given. In the resource-restricted settings in which we practice, there are apparently many multidrug resistant tuberculosis patients with a limited number of these having laboratory back-up. Over 50 such patients have undergone sputum culture study for AFB and have shown interesting multidrug resistant patterns. In the majority of these cases it is not possible to offer second-line drugs due to financial constraints and lack of compliance. There are instances of recovery from resistant tuberculosis in a selected number of patients who can afford antiretroviral therapy and who have been significantly benefited.

Bacterial Pneumonia

One of the causes of prolonged fever and cough is bacterial pneumonia. This could be either lobar pneumonia or, rarely, bilateral pneumonia. Lobar pneumonia is caused by pyogenic bacteria, while bilateral pneumonia is mostly caused by gram negative organisms. Quite often the patient is toxic and has septicaemia. In resource-restricted settings it is advisable to start treatment empirically without awaiting for a microbiology report. It is preferable to use adequately higher generation antibiotics combinations capable of covering a wider range of micro-organisms.

Pneumocystis Carinii Pneumonia (PCP) Infection

Initially tuberculosis accounted for most chest infections, but as the HIV/AIDS epidemic has reached maturity in India, detection of PCP has become fairly common, provided there is a high index of suspicion amongst heath-care providers. More than 10 per cent of chest infections reveal co-infection with pulmonary tuberculosis and PCP. Besides typical presentations of PCP, for example fever, cough, breathlessness on exertion, cyanosis, chest X-ray showing paracardiac haziness and HRCT chest showing ground glass opacity in the lung fields, there are also unusual presentations such as productive cough, absence of fever, a chest X-ray that may appear normal, HRCT chest that may appear normal. Careful sputum examination may identify PCP in cystic or trophozoite forms in a proportion of patients, depending on the severity of infection. However, the direct immunofluorescence test is confirmatory and supplementary. In a few patients where arterial gases were studied they revealed proportionate abnormalities, especially low pO^2 level. Few of our patients showed advanced PCP disease on chest X-ray mimicking gram negative pneumonia. The laboratory results of PCP identification revealed that the routine sputum collected by bronchial lavage is superior to hypertonic saline nebulisation, which is superior to routinely coughed sputum. We practice treating PCP using induction therapy with oral cotrimoxazole double strength two tablets three times a day for at least three weeks followed by life-long secondary prophylaxis using daily one double strength tablet. In patients who get breathlessness on exertion or who have low pO^2, systemic steroid therapy is significantly useful. None of our 590 PCP patients showed allergy to sulpha; however clindamycin combined with primaquine is an available alternative but is expensive. We have observed that over 10 per cent of PCP patients relapse within three months; therefore we understand that induction therapy of three weeks should be only tapered provided sputum has become negative for PCP during a follow-up study. We do not know whether we also experience cotrimoxazole-resistant PCP infection. Fifteen per cent of patients developed PCP infection in spite of receiving primary prophylaxis with daily one double strength cotrimoxazole or in spite of receiving triple drug antiretroviral therapy.

Miscellaneous chest infections include fungal and viral infection. In sick and wasted patients with advanced HIV disease, we have seen extensive bilateral pulmonary infiltration and nodular opacities suggestive of polymicrobial etiology; given empirically antibiotic, antifungal and antituberculous drugs these patients show reasonable recovery. In our experience candidiasis, aspergillosis, cryptococcosis and histoplasosis are etiological organsitions for fungal chest infections. We have picked up cytomegalovirus pneumonia only on autopsy study.

The treatment for opportunistic infections is subsidised in public hospitals in India; the treatment for tuberculosis and PCP, however, are totally free. Despite this, compliance with treatment is unsatisfactory. The only way to ensure satisfactory compliance is to offer strong counselling services to HIV-positive individuals. Currently, the counselling services are grossly inadequate. Initiation of directly observed therapy (DOT) for tuberculosis is needed. Early recognition and prompt and adequate treatment of individual opportunistic infection will avoid further damage to the body's immune system, induce a sense of well-being and preserve productivity, thereby maintaining socio-economic status. This will also help to prevent morbidity and mortality due to OIs.

HIV Treatment and Care

Antiretroviral treatment options are still prohibitively expensive. Only 3 to 5 per cent of HIV-infected individuals can currently afford antiretroviral therapy.[10] Because of the perceived incurable nature of HIV infection, ignorance, advertisements in the various media promoting cures for HIV/AIDS, myths about lack of side-effects of allopathic medicine and inability to afford the cost of modern anti-retroviral drugs, the use of alternative or traditional medicines is very popular among HIV-infected people. In India, zidovudine, stavudine, lamivudine, saquinavir, retonavir, nevirapine and zalcitabine are available locally at nearly 60 per cent of international cost, while the remaining antiretroviral drugs need to be imported at standard international cost. There is no subsidised programme available for antiretroviral therapy in India. The individual patient has to bear the total cost. Even health insurance does not cover treatment cost for HIV-positive individuals. It is important to offer intensive counselling to patients wanting to start antiretroviral therapy (ART), stressing the pill burden, duration of therapy, likely side-effects due to therapy, importance of adherence to therapy, limitations of benefits of therapy, possibilities of drug interactions between ART and other drugs used for treatment of OIs. In our personal experience, in spite of intensive counselling services, due to the lack of initiatives, financial burden, inability to bear side-effects of ART, pill burden and sometime non-availability of ART, the compliance rate is only 40 per cent. There is constant danger of developing significant resistance to individual antiretroviral agents. There is lack of adequate knowledge and skill in using antiretroviral therapy amongst treating physicians, which also contributes to the failure of ART.

In India, as in other parts of the world, the HIV epidemic has created significant social challenges.[13] The stigma attached to the disease is immense and includes irrational fears held by members of the various health professions. AIDS awareness is increasing among urban youth, but it is much lower in the rural areas. Several non-governmental organisations are working on developing effective communication tools to reach the general population.

References

1. Simoes, E A F, Babu, P G, Jeyakumari, H M and John, T J (1987). 'The initial detection of human immunodeficiency virus 1 and its subsequent spread in prostitutes in Tamil Nadu, India', *AIDS* 6: 1030–4.

2. Bollinger, R C, Tripathy, S P and Quinn, T C (1995). 'The human immunodeficiency virus epidemic in India. Current magnitude and future projections', *Medicine* (Baltimore) 74: 97–106.

3. Sarkar, S, Mookerjee, P, Roy, A, Naik, TN, Singh, JK, Sharma, AR, Singh, PK, Tripathy, SP and Pal, SC (1991). 'Descriptive epidemiology of intravenous heroin users – a new risk group for transmission of HIV in India', *J Infect* 23: 201–7.

4. Joshi, PL, Prasada Rao, JVR (1999). 'Changing epidemiology of HIV/AIDS in India', *AIDS Research & Review* 2: 1–7.

5. Kumar, S (1999). 'India has the largest number of people infected with HIV', *Lancet*, 353: 48.

6. Talib, SH, Bansal, MP and Kamble, MM (1993). 'HIV-1 seropositivity in pulmonary tuberculosis (a study of 340 cases from Marathwada), India', *J Pathol Microbiology* 36: 383–8.

7. Jujar, S, Maniar, JK and Saple, DG (1998). Compliance of Tuberculosis patients in HIV/AIDS Clinic G.T.Hospital, Mumbai, India, Int Conf AIDS, 12:292 (abstract no. 22151).

8. Maniar, J, Saple, DG and Kurimura, T (1998). Changing pattern of opportunistic infections, Int Conf AIDS 12:135 (abstract no. 13245).

9. Maniar, J and Hira, S. Clinical spectrum of HIV in Bombay, Int Conf AIDS, 10(1):154 (abstract no. PB 0042).

10. Saple, D and Maniar, JK (1998). Scenario of antiretroviral therapy (ART) in 25000 HIV/AIDS individuals in Mumbai, India, Int Conf AIDS, 12:345 (abstract no. 22406).

11. Desai, Swati, Saple, DG and Maniar, JK (1998). Chemoprophylaxis for TB in HIV/AIDS, Mumbai, Int Conf AIDS, 1166 (abstract no. 60907).

12. Subir, Kumar Dey, Pal, NKP, Bhattacharjee, NB and Pal, GP (1998). Spectrum of HIV infection in tuberculosis – urban and rural experience of different perspectives, West Bengal, India, 12th World AIDS Conf 292 (abstract no. 22152).

13. Dietrich, U, Maniar, JK, and Rubsamen-Walgmann, H (1995). 'The epidemiology of AIDS in India', *Trend Microbiol* 3.17.2.

14. Maniar, JK and Saple, DG (1998). 'The HIV/AIDS epidemic in India', *HIV & AIDS current trends* 4:3: 3–6.

Contributors

John Anderson is a member of the Commonwealth Association of Planners and BEPIC.

Lalit K Bhutani MD FRCP (Edin) was formerly Dean and Director of the All India Institute of Medical Sciences, New Delhi, India. Dr Bhutani worked as a Professor and Head of the Department of Dermatology and Venereology for 26 years before his retirement from the Institute. He has served as a short-term consultant with various organisations, including WHO, SIDA, DIFD and the British Council, on programmes related to HIV/AIDS and STDs. He was a member of the WHO teams evaluating Sonagachi and Bombay Sexual Healthcare projects.

Dr Lalit K Bhutani
Sitaram Bhartia Institute of Science and Research
B-16 Mehrauli Institutional Area
New Delhi 110016, India
E-mail: sbisr@vsnl.com
lbhutani@hotmail.com

Dr Prakash Bora
5719/212, Shivan, opp Odeon
R. Narkar Marg, Pantnagar
Ghatkopar (East)
Mumbai-400075
India
Tel: 91 22 5165 893
Fax: 91 22 5163 590
E-mail: pcbora18@yahoo.com

Ian Campbell, a physician and Salvation Army officer, is the International Health Programme Consultant of the Salvation Army International Headquarters. This task includes facilitation of participatory design and evaluation of home- and community-based approaches to a range of health issues, often resourced by hospitals or clinic systems.

Usuf Chikte BChD (UWC), DHSM (Wits), MChD (Wits), MSc (Lon) is Head and Chief Specialist, Department of Community Dentistry, University of Stellenbosch, Tygerberg, South Africa.

Professor Usuf Chikte
Department of Community Dentistry
University of Stellenbosch
Private Bag X1
Tygerberg 7505
South Africa
Tel: 21-937 3149
Fax: 21-931 2287
e-mail: umec@maties.sun.ac.za

Carol Coombe has worked in Africa since she went to Zambia as a CUSO volunteer in 1968. From 1985–1994 she was based at the Commonwealth Secretariat Education Department, latterly as Chief Programme Officer and first Convenor of the ADEA Working Group on the Teaching Profession. Since the 1994 election in South Africa, she has worked as an independent advisor to agencies and governments in the SADC region, principally on educator development and support, and management issues. In this context she has become increasingly concerned about the impact of HIV/AIDS on management, human resources and sector development in Africa.

Carol Coombe,
Education Advisor
184 Lisdogan Ave
Pretoria 0083
South Africa
Tel: (27) (12) 342 2857
Fax: (27) (12) 342 6320
E-mail: coombe@mweb.co.za

Monica Dolan
Monica Dolan
AIDS Section
International Division
CAFOD

Ian Douglas is the Chairman of the Board of Governors, Commonwealth Human Ecology Council.

José Esparza is the Co-ordinator of the recently established HIV Vaccine Initiative, jointly co-sponsored by WHO and UNAIDS, in Geneva, Switzerland. Dr Esparza obtained his MD degree at Zulia University in Maracaibo, Venezuela and a PhD degree in Virology and Epidemiology at Baylor College of Medicine in Houston, Texas, USA. He was Professor of Virology and Chair of the Centre for Microbiology and Cell Biology at the Venezuelan Institute of Scientific Research in Caracas, Venezuela. He was a Visiting Professor at the Department of Microbiology and Immunology at Duke University Medical Centre in Durham, North Carolina, USA, and is an Associate Professor at the Virus Research Centre, University of Quebec, Montreal, Canada. Dr Esparza joined WHO in 1986, first with the Division of Communicable Diseases and then with the Global Programme on AIDS (GPA), where he was the Chief of the Vaccine Development Unit. From 1996 to 1999 he was Leader of the UNAIDS Vaccine Team.

Dr Jose Esparza
Co-ordinator, WHO-UNAIDS HIV
Vaccine Initiative
20 Avenue Appia
CH-1211 Geneva 27
Switzerland
Tel: 900 41 22 791 4392
Fax: 900 41 22 791 4741
E-mail: esparzaj@unaids.org

Martin Foreman
Director, AIDS Programme
Panos Institute
9 White Lion Street
London N1 9PD, UK
Tel: + 44 20 7239 7604
Fax: + 44 20 7278 0345
E-mail: martinf@panoslondon.org.uk

Dorothy Garland began a long and utterly absorbing involvement, in an administrative capacity, with the universities of the Commonwealth soon after graduating in Modern Languages. For 12 years she represented in London the interests of at first just one, and subsequently all, of the Nigerian Federal Universities, witnessing the huge growth in that system in the years 1972–1984. For the past 15 years she has worked for the Association of Commonwealth Universities, where she is now Deputy Secretary General and Director of External Relations.

Dorothy Garland
Director of External Relations and
Deputy Secretary General
Association of Commonwealth
Universities
36 Gordon Square
London WC1H UP, UK
Tel: +44 (0) 171 387 8572
Fax: +44 (0) 171 387 2655
E-mail d.garland@acu.ac.uk

David Hall is Science Advisor to the Commonwealth Human Ecology Council.

Andrew Hobbs
20 Broadgate, Preston
Lancashire PR1 8DX
United Kingdom
E-mail: andhobbs@btinternet.com

John Hubley has extensive experience working with AIDS control programmes in more than 15 countries in Africa, Asia, the Pacific and Europe. He has worked with WHO as a consultant both in AIDS and other health topics. He is author of *The AIDS Handbook* and *Communicating Health*, together with a number of other books and papers on AIDS and health promotion. He now divides his time between freelance work as a consultant/author and a teaching post at Leeds Metropolitan University where he is

Senior Lecturer in Health Promotion and Health Education. His main research interest is in the evaluation of health education and health promotion in developing countries and the Leeds Health Education Database Project.

Dr John Hubley
21 Arncliffe Road
Leeds LS16 5AP, UK
Fax: 0113 2305 224
E-mail: john@hubley.co.uk

Michael Jacino
Partnerships and Marketing Development Advisor
HIV/AIDS Policy
Co-ordination and Programmes Division
Health Canada.

Dr Elly Katabira is a co-founder of TASO, physician and Senior Lecturer.

Dr Elly Katabira,
Mulago Hospital, Medical School,
Makerere University,
P.O. Box 7062 Kampala,
Uganda.
E-mail katabira@imul.comv

Dr Neena Khanna is currently working as an Associate Professor in the Department of Dermatology and Venereology at the All India Institute of Medical Sciences, New Delhi, India.

Richard Mambwe
c/o Project Concern International
PO Box32320
Lusaka
Zambia
E-mail: pci@zamnet.zm

Professor Janak K. Maniar, MBBS DVD, DDV, MD (Skin and STD) is Honorary Professor of Dermatology and STDs at Grant Medical College, University of Bombay. He was the Organising Secretary for the First National Conference on

AIDS held in Bombay in 1993 and served as a member of the International Advisory Board for the World Congress on STD/AIDS, held in Singapore in 1995. He was Chairman of the Annual National Conference of Indian Associations of STDs and AIDS held in Bombay in 1998 and has also served as Chairman of the National Conference on Perinatal HIV and Paediatric AIDS, in Bombay during 1998 and 1999.

Professor Maniar has worked in the field of HIV/AIDS medicine in Bombay since 1986 and has been actively involved in the management of HIV/AIDS patients. He was the first Asian physician to detect the existence of HIV-2 infection in Asia-Pacific in December 1990, in collaboration with a German virology laboratory unit. He was also the first Asian physician to detect HIV-1 subtype C. Professor Maniar has written numerous papers and delivered many conference presentations.

Professor Janak Maniar
Department of Dermatovenereology and AIDS Medicine
G.T. Hosptial
Grant Medical College
Bombay, India
Fax: 91-22-208 3184 / 91-22-208 2847
E-mail: jkmaniar@bom5.vsnl.net.in

Winnie Mpanju-Shumbusho is currently the Director of the HIV/AIDS/STD Initiative of WHO in Geneva. She obtained her MD and Master of Medicine degrees from the University of Dar-es-Salaam, Tanzania, and a Master of Public Health degree from Tulane University in New Orleans, Louisiana, USA. Before joining WHO, Dr Mpanju-Shumbusho worked at the Commonwealth Regional Health Community Secretariat (CRHCS) for East, Central and Southern Africa (ECSA) in various capacities, including serving as the Regional Secretary and

Head of Mission, Co-ordinator of the Reproductive Health Programme and Assistant Co-ordinator of the Health Research Programme. Prior to this she served as the Head of the Department of Community Health at the Institute of Public Health, Muhimbili University College of Health Sciences, University of Dar-es-Salaam, where she was also a lecturer in Community Health as well as Paediatrics and Child Health. She has also served as a Technical Adviser to the ECSA Ministries of Health and as a consultant for various international organisations.

Dr Winnie K Mpanju-Shumbusho
Director, HIV/AIDS/STD Initiative
WHO
20 Avenue Appia
CH-1211 Geneva
Switzerland

Dr Francis Mubiru, who was in charge of the HIV clinic of TASO in Mulago Hospital and contributed to this article, unfortunately died in a traffic accident in Uganda shortly after the article was written.

Mary Lyn Mulvihill
Partnerships and Marketing Consultant
HIV/AIDS Policy, Co-ordination and
Programmes Division
Health Canada.
E-mail: Mary_Lyn_Mulvihill@hc-sc.gc.ca

Dr Sudeshni Naidoo BDS (Lon),
LDS.RCS (Eng), MDPH (Lon),
DDPH.RCS (Eng), MChD (UWC),
Department of Community Dentistry,
University of Stellenbosch, Tygerberg,
South Africa.

Dr Eric van Praag is a medical officer and health planner.

Dr Eric van Praag, Director HIV Care,
Family Health International,

2101 Wilson Boulevard, Suite 700,
Arlington VA 22201, USA
Tel: 1 703 516 9779
Fax: 1 703 516 9781
E-mail: evanpraag@fhi.org

Regina Cammy Shakakata
Tel: 091 240247 (or) 1 321 733 9314
Fax: 1 321 733 9160
E-mail: shakakatar@whoafr.org

Margaret Sills has worked as a freelance health promotion specialist since 1980 and spent 18 months working in the Health Department of the Commonwealth Secretariat. She now works at King's College, London where she teaches on the Master's Programme in Health Promotion and Health Education and is the Academic Director for the Learning and Teaching Support Network: Health Sciences and Practice Centre.

Ann Smith
AIDS Section
International Division
CAFOD

Annie Watson is the Director of the Commonwealth Trade Union Council.

Alan Whiteside is Associate Professor and Director of the Health Economics and HIV/AIDS Research Division, University of Natal, Durban, South Africa.

Professor Alan Whiteside
Director, Health Economics and
HIV/AIDS Research Division
University of Natal
Durban
South Africa
Tel: 27 31 260 2592
Fax: 27 31 260 2587
E-mail: whitesid@shep.und.ac.za